Handbook of Epilepsy

Acquisitions Editor: Mark Placito
Developmental Editor: Mattie Bialer
Manufacturing Manager: Dennis Teston
Production Manager: Maxine Langweil
Cover Designer: Jeane Norton
Indexer: Alexandra Nickerson
Compositor: Lippincott-Raven Electronic Production
Printer: R. R. Donnelly

Printed in the United States of America

9 8 7 6 5 4 3 2 1

Library of Congress Cataloging-in-Publication Data

Browne, Thomas R.
    Handbook of epilepsy / Thomas R. Browne, Gregory L. Holmes.
        p.   cm.
    Includes bibliographical references and index.
    ISBN 0-316-11053-1 (Alk. paper)
    1. Epilepsy—Handbooks, manuals, etc.   2. Epilepsy in children—
Handbooks, manuals, etc.   I. Holmes, Gregory L.   II. Title.
    [DNLM: 1. Epilepsy—handbooks.   WL 39 B884h 1997]
    RC372.B76   1997
    616.8953—dc21
    DNLM/DLC
    for Library of Congress   97-10478
                                                                         CIP

To Cesare T. Lombroso, M.D.
Mentor, Colleague, Friend.

Contents

Preface

The purpose of this book is to provide concise, up-to-date, and clinically oriented reviews of each of the major areas in the diagnosis and management of epilepsy. In meeting this purpose we faced two challenges. The first challenge was to present the material in a volume of proper size for practicing physicians. Through careful selection and editing of the most clinically relevant information, we have strived to cover the field of epilepsy concisely without "dumbing down" the content. Select, recent and comprehensive references on all important topics are provided. Using these references and computer literature search programs, the reader should be able to go into a topic in a comprehensive fashion if desired.

The second challenge was dealing with the International Classification of the Epilepsies in a concise and clinically relevant manner. This classification is large, complex and potentially confusing. On the other hand, the classification contains much useful and recent information of clinical relevance. We have elected to group the epilepsies by age of onset. This grouping reduces the differential diagnostic possibilities to a manageable size for a given patient and provides the physician with an overview of the possible syndromes to consider in a patient of a given age.

To effectively manage patients with epilepsy, it is necessary to have a clear understanding of the differential diagnosis of the various types of seizures and types of epilepsy, the spectrum and uses of available antiepileptic drugs, the clinical pharmacology of antiepileptic drugs, and the spectrum and uses of nonpharmacologic therapy. All of the basic information on these topics is contained in this book. The physician who masters this information will provide quality care for patients with epilepsy and will find managing such patients interesting and rewarding.

EPILEPSY: DEFINITIONS AND BACKGROUND

I. DEFINITION OF EPILEPSY

Hippocrates recognized epilepsy as an organic process of the brain. However, many ancient writers considered seizures to be the work of supernatural forces. In fact, the word epilepsy comes from a Greek word meaning "to be seized by forces from without."

J.H. Jackson gave direction to the understanding of epilepsy in the late 19th century by carefully analyzing individual cases. From his observations, Jackson (10) formulated the modern definition of epilepsy: "an occasional, excessive, and disorderly discharge of nerve tissue." Jackson further concluded: "This discharge occurs in all degrees; it occurs with all sorts of conditions of ill health at all ages, and under innumerable circumstances." His emphasis on the clinical description of a seizure, beginning with the mode of onset, led to the concept of focal epilepsy with subsequent spread of discharging cells.

Epilepsy is a complex symptom caused by a variety of pathologic processes in the brain. It is characterized by occasional (paroxysmal), excessive, and disorderly discharging of neurons, which can be detected by clinical manifestations, electroencephalographic (EEG) recording, or both. Paroxysmal discharges of neurons occur when the threshold for firing of the neuronal membranes is reduced beyond the capability of intrinsic membrane–threshold-stabilizing mechanisms to prevent firing (see Section V, below). The attack may be localized and remain restricted in its focus, or it can spread to other areas of the brain. When the size of the discharging area is sufficient, a clinical seizure occurs; otherwise, it may be limited to localized, asymptomatic electrical disturbances. The particular site of the brain affected determines the clinical expression of the seizure. When the synchronized discharges of a neuronal population are recorded by an EEG from the scalp, the paroxysms appear as spikes, slow waves, and spike-wave potentials.

For the patient with epilepsy, the disorder is defined in more personal terms. Among the factors that define epilepsy for the individual are: what he/she experiences or recalls about the experience; what others around him/her observe and describe; the frequency and duration of attacks; and the impact on self-image and social adjustment.

II. PARTS OF A SEIZURE

The period during which the seizure actually occurs is defined as the *ictus* or *ictal period*. The *aura* is the earliest portion of a seizure recognized, and the only part remembered by the patient; it may act as a "warning." The time immediately following a seizure is referred to as the *postical period*. The interval between seizures is the *interictal period*.

III. TYPES OF EPILEPTIC SEIZURES AND TYPES OF EPILEPSY: CLASSIFICATIONS

There are two types of classifications used for epilepsy: (1) classifications of the epileptic seizures and (2) classifications of the epilepsies. Classifications of epileptic seizures are concerned with classifying each individual seizure as a single event, based upon clinical and EEG information. Classifications of the epilepsies are designed to classify syndromes in which the type or types of seizure(s) are one, but not the only, feature of the syndrome. Other features such as etiology, age of onset, and evidence of brain pathology are also included in classifications of the epilepsies.

The classification of epileptic seizures used throughout this book is the most recent revision (1981) of the Clinical and Electroencephalographic Classification of Epileptic Seizures of the International League Against Epilepsy ("International Classification of Epileptic Seizures") (3). The classification of the epilepsies used is the most recent revision (1989) of the Classification of Epilepsies and Epileptic Syndromes of the International League Against Epilepsy ("International Classification of Epilepsies") (4). These classifications are now used by most experts.

A. International Classification of Epileptic Seizures

The International Classification of Epileptic Seizures is summarized in Table 1-1 and presented in detail in Table 2-1. Seizures are first classified into two broad categories: (a) partial seizures (seizure beginning in a relatively small location in the brain) and (b) generalized seizures (seizures that are bilaterally symmetrical and without local onset). Seizures are then further classified depending on the exact clinical and EEG manifestations of the seizure. A summary of the clinical manifestations of the

Table 1-1. *Summary of international classification of epileptic seizures*

I. Partial (Focal, Local) Seizures
- A. Simple partial seizures (consciousness not impaired)
- B. Complex partial seizures (temporal lobe or psychomotor seizures; consciousness impaired)
- C. Partial seizures evolving to secondarily generalized seizures [tonic-clonic (grand mal), tonic or clonic]

II. Generalized seizures (convulsive or nonconvulsive)
- A. Absence (petit mal) seizures
- B. Myoclonic seizures
- C. Tonic seizures
- D. Atonic seizures
- E. Clonic seizures
- F. Tonic-clonic (grand mal) seizures

III. Unclassified epileptic seizures (caused by incomplete data)

Modified from Commission on Classification and Terminology of the International League Against Epilepsy. Proposal for revised clinical and electroencephalographic classification of epileptic seizures. *Epilepsia* 1981;22:489–501, with permission.

principal types of epileptic seizures recognized by the International Classification of Epileptic Seizures is presented below. For a complete description of the clinical and EEG features of each seizure type, see Chapter 2.

1. Simple Partial (Focal) Seizures

Simple partial seizures are caused by a local cortical discharge, which results in seizure symptoms appropriate to the function of the discharging area of the brain *without impairment of consciousness*. Simple partial seizures may consist of motor, sensory, autonomic, or psychic signs or symptoms, or combinations of these (see Chapter 2).

2. Complex Partial (Psychomotor, Temporal Lobe) Seizures

The crucial distinction between simple partial seizures and complex partial seizures is that *consciousness is impaired* in the latter and not in the former. Impaired consciousness is defined as the inability to respond normally to exogenous stimuli owing to the altered awareness or responsiveness.

At the onset of a complex partial seizure, any of the symptoms or signs (motor, sensory, autonomic, or psychic) of a simple partial seizure may occur without impairment of consciousness, providing an aura. The central feature of the complex partial seizure is impairment of consciousness, which may occur with or without a preceding simple partial aura. There may be no other symptoms or

Table 1-2. *Summary of international classification of epilepsies and epilepsy syndromes (with age of onset)*

1.1 Localization related/idiopathic epilepsies
  *Benign childhood epilepsy with centrotemporal spikes (C)
  *Childhood epilepsy with occipital paroxysms (C)
1.2 Localization related/symptomatic epilepsies
  *Temporal lobe, *frontal lobe, *parietal lobe, or
  *occipital lobe (I, C or A)
2.1 Generalized/idiopathic epilepsies
  *Benign familial neonatal seizures (N)
  *Benign neonatal convulsions (N)
  *Benign myoclonic epilepsy in infancy (C)
  *Childhood absence epilepsy (C)
  *Juvenile absence epilepsy (C or A)
  *Juvenile myoclonic epilepsy (C or A)
  *Epilepsy with tonic-clonic seizures on awakening (C or A)
  *Epilepsy with random tonic-clonic seizures (C or A)
2.2 Generalized/symptomatic epilepsies
  *West syndrome (infantile spasms) (I)
  *Lennox Gastaut syndrome (C)
2.3 Generalized/either idiopathic or symptomatic epilepsies
  *Benign myoclonic epilepsy of infancy (I)
  *Severe myoclonic epilepsy of infancy (I)
  *Myoclonic-astatic epilepsy (I)
  *Progressive myoclonic seizures (C or A)
3. Both localization related and generalized epilepsies
  *Neonatal seizures (N)
4. Situation-related epilepsies
  *Febrile convulsions (I, C)
  *Alcohol-related (A)
  *Drug-related (A)
  *Eclampsia (A)
  *Seizures with specific modes of precipitation (reflex epilepsies) (C or A)

---

*Specific epilepsy syndrome.
N, neonatal (birth–2 months); I, infancy (2–12 months); C, childhood (1–12 years); A, juvenile and adults (12 years and older).
Modified from reference (4) with permission.

signs during the period of impaired consciousness, or there may be *automatisms* (i.e., unconscious acts that are "automatic" and of which the patient has no recollection). The attack characteristically ends gradually, with a period of postictal drowsiness or confusion (see Chapter 2).

3. Absence (Petit Mal) Seizures

Absence seizures consist of sudden onset and cessation of impaired responsiveness, accompanied by a unique 3-Hz spike-and-wave EEG pattern. There is no aura and little or no postictal symptomatology. The majority of absence seizures last 10 sec or less and may be accompanied by mild clonic components, atonic or tonic components, automatisms, or autonomic components. Absence seizures usually begin between the ages of 5 and 12 years and often stop spontaneously in the teens (see Chapter 2).

4. Myoclonic Seizures

Myoclonic seizures consist of brief, sudden muscle contractions that may be generalized or localized, symmetric or asymmetric, synchronous or asynchronous. There is usually no detectable loss of consciousness (see Chapter 2).

5. Tonic Seizures

Tonic seizures consist of a sudden increase in muscle tone in the axial or extremity muscles, or both, producing a number of characteristic postures. Consciousness is usually partially or completely lost. Prominent autonomic phenomena occur. Postictal alteration of consciousness is usually brief, but may last several minutes. Tonic seizures are relatively rare and usually begin between 1 and 7 years of age (see Chapter 2).

6. Atonic Seizures

Atonic seizures consist of sudden loss of muscle tone. The loss of muscle tone may be confined to a group of muscles, such as the neck, resulting in a head drop. Alternatively, atonic seizures may involve all trunk muscles, leading to a fall to the ground (see Chapter 2).

7. Clonic Seizures

Clonic seizures occur almost exclusively in early childhood. The attack begins with loss or impairment of consciousness associated with sudden hypotonia or a brief, generalized tonic spasm. This is followed by one to several minutes of bilateral jerks, which are often asymmetric and may predominate in one limb. During the attack there may be great variability in the amplitude, frequency, and spatial distribution of these jerks from moment to moment. In other children, particularly those aged 1 to 3 years, the jerks remain bilateral and synchronous throughout the attack. Postictally there may be rapid recovery or a prolonged period of confusion or coma (see Chapter 2).

8. Tonic-Clonic (Grand Mal) Seizures

Before the tonic phase there may be bilateral jerks of the extremities or focal seizure activity. The onset of the

INCIDENCE PER 100,000

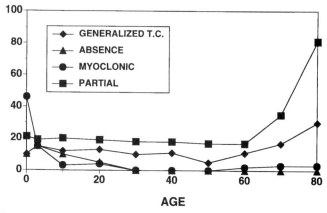

AGE

Fig. 1-2. Incidence rates of epilepsy by seizure type from Rochester, Minnesota, 1935–1979. From ref. (1) with permission.

Incidence is the occurrence of new cases of epilepsy per unit of person-time. Incidence of epilepsy is usually estimated at 30 to 50 per 100,000 person-years. Incidence can also be reported by clinical seizure type (see Fig. 1-2).

Note in Figs. 1-1 and 1-2 that the prevalence and cumulative incidence of epilepsy, and the incidence of partial seizures, increase dramatically in the elderly. This will be discussed in more detail in Chapter 13.

V. BASIC MECHANISMS OF EPILEPSY

Epilepsy is a paroxysmal disorder characterized by abnormal neuronal discharges. While the causes of epilepsy are many, the fundamental disorder is secondary to abnormal synchronous discharges of a network of neurons. Epilepsy can be secondary to either abnormal neuronal membranes or an imbalance between excitatory and inhibitory influences.

In this section, we will first review basic principles of generation and cessation of seizure activity: excitation and inhibition of neuronal membranes, excitation and inhibition of neurons by neurotransmitters, generation of EEG potentials, generation of interictal discharges, generation of seizure activity, and cessation of seizure activity. Specific seizure types are created by excitation and inhibition in specific neuronal networks, and this will be reviewed for partial seizures and absence seizures in the second part of this section.

A. Principles of Generation and Cessation of Seizure Activity

1. Excitation and Inhibition of Neuronal Membranes

Neuronal membranes consist of lipid bilayers mixed with proteins that traverse the membrane and form ion channels. Each neuron has a resting potential that represents the voltage difference between the inside and outside of the cell. This potential difference exists because of the separation of positive and negative changes across the cell membrane. The extracellular space along the membrane is dominated by sodium (Na^+) and chloride (Cl^-) ions, while potassium (K^+), proteins, and organic acids are found in the intracellular space. Membranes are permeable to Na^+, Cl^-, and K^+, but impermeable to large organic ions and proteins. Because the lipid bilayers act as a barrier to the diffusion of ions, a net excess of positive charges outside and negative charges inside produces a *resting membrane potential* of approximately -50 to -80 mV.

Ion leaks across the membrane occur moving from high concentration to low concentration: Na^+ leaks in and K^+ out. With time, the inside and outside concentration (across the membrane) may change. The Na^+–K^+ pump extrudes Na^+ from the cell and brings in K^+, counterbalancing the leakage. The pump, which moves Na^+ and K^+ against their net electrochemical gradients, requires energy that is derived from hydrolysis of adenosine triphosphate (ATP). A reduction in the negativity of this polarized state is called *depolarization*; an increase in the negativity of the resting potential is known as *hyperpolarization*. Membrane permeability changes that allow Na^+ to enter the cell lead to depolarization, while membrane changes that allow K^+ to exit the cell or Cl^- to enter the cell, result in hyperpolarization. If there is a sufficient decrease in intracellular negativity, an action potential is generated (Fig. 1-3).

2. Excitation and Inhibition of Neurons by Neurotransmitters

Protein segments extend out of the membrane and serve as receptor sites. *Ionotropic receptors* directly alter the conductance of the ion channel when bound to a neurotransmitter. Examples of ionotropic receptors include the gamma-aminobutyric acid ($GABA_A$) receptors that increase Cl^- conductance and the NMDA receptors which increase the permeability to Na^+. Neurotransmitters (such as GABA) that cause hyperpolarization of the neuron give rise to *inhibitory postsynaptic potentials* (IPSPs), which result in a greater intracellular negativity than

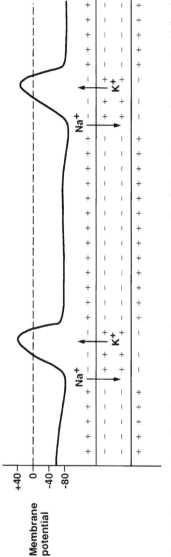

Fig. 1-3. Propagation of action potential along axon as a result of changing membrane potentials. At rest the inside of the neuron is negative compared with the extracellular space. An action potential is generated during transient breakdown in gradient between K⁺ and Na⁺ ions. From ref. (8), with permission.

baseline. Neurotransmitters that lead to depolarization (such as excitatory amino acids) give rise to excitatory postsynaptic potentials, which result in an inward flow of positive charges through the synaptic membrane, leaving a relatively negative extracellular environment. Whether a neuron generates an action potential is determined by the relative balance of EPSPs and IPSPs. Figure 1-4 demonstrates current flow with EPSPs and IPSPs.

A second type of neurotransmitter receptor is the *metabatropic receptor*. When a transmitter binds to the metabatropic receptor, it activates a *second messenger system* (G-protein: guanyl nucleotide-binding protein). The activated G-protein may then open an ion channel or activate an enzyme, such as a cyclase (cyclic AMP) or hydrolase, to affect the generation of additional messenger molecules within a cell. Examples of receptors that activate second messenger systems include $GABA_B$ receptors, peptide and catecholaminergic receptors, as well as the metabatropic receptors activated by glutamate. Note that $GABA_A$ receptors are ionotropic receptors that enhance chloride conductance, while $GABA_B$ receptors are metabatropic receptors that are coupled through G-proteins to calcium or potassium ion channels.

3. Generation of EEG Potentials

The EEG is based on volume conduction of ionic currents generated by nerve cells through the extracellular space. Recorded EEG potentials arise from extracellular current flow from summated EPSPs and IPSPs. The EEG does not record activity from single neurons, but is dependent on the summation of thousands to millions of postsynaptic potentials (PSPs) and, therefore, represents activity from a large neuronal aggregation. While nerve action potentials have higher voltage changes than EPSPs and IPSPs, the lack of summation and short duration of the action potentials adds little to EEG activity.

4. Generation of Interictal Discharges

The hallmark of the epileptic neuron in experimental models of epilepsy is membrane depolarization. During an interictal discharge, the cell membrane near the soma undergoes a relatively high voltage (approximately 10–15 mV) and relatively long (100–200 msec) depolarization associated with bursts of spike activity (Fig. 1-5). This depolarization is much longer than the depolarization seen with EPSPs, which is in the range of 10 to 16 msec. The long depolarization has the effect of generating a

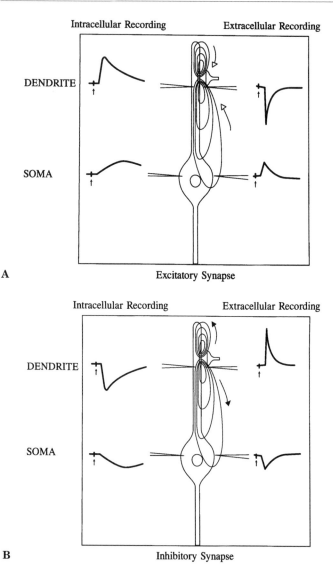

Intracellular Recording   Extracellular Recording

DENDRITE

SOMA

A   Excitatory Synapse

Intracellular Recording   Extracellular Recording

DENDRITE

SOMA

B   Inhibitory Synapse

Fig. 1-4. A: Example of current flow as a result of EPSP on the apical dendrites. B: Example of current flow as a result of IPSP on the apical dendrites. From ref. (10), with permission.

ment of generalized seizures. Once the enhanced sensitivity has developed, the effect is long-lasting and the animal can be classified as kindled. Kindling is not limited to the original kindling agent, but may result in increased seizure susceptibility to other kindling agents. Kindling is now widely accepted as an animal model of partial epilepsy.

In the kindling model there are three mechanisms that underlie the development of partial seizures. First, there is evidence of enhanced NMDA receptor-mediated transmission in dentate granule cells. This suggests that excitatory input into the hippocampus will be heightened in the dentate. A second mechanism is the loss of hilar neurons which normally activate inhibitory basket cells. Loss of these hilar neurons leads to loss of inhibition of dentate granule cells and increased hippocampal excitation. The third mechanism in kindling is the synaptic reorganization of granule-cell excitatory cell output. Following kindling, it has been noted that there is an aberrant growth of granule-cell axons (called mossy fibers) back into the inner molecular layer of the dentate. The spouting of mossy-fiber axons is readily observed with the Timm method, a histochemical technique that selectively stains mossy-fiber axon terminals because of their high zinc content. Since the neurotransmitter of the mossy fibers is presumably glutamate, these aberrant synaptic conditions may contribute to the state of hyperexcitability that either provokes or facilitates abnormal discharges. The net effect of such synaptic reorganization has been shown to be excitatory in the kindling model.

2. Absence Seizures

The observation that 3-Hz spike-and-wave discharges in absence seizures appear simultaneously and synchronously in all electrode locations, led early investigators to speculate that the pathophysiologic mechanisms of absence seizures must involve "deep" structures with widespread connections between the two hemispheres (see Figs. 2-2 and 6-3). A number of studies have recently suggested that the basic underlying mechanism in absence seizures involves thalamocortical circuitry and the generation of abnormal oscillatory rhythms in the neuronal network. Studies in animals and *in vitro* have now demonstrated this neuronal circuit that generates the oscillatory thalamocortical burst-firing observed during absence seizures (Fig. 1-7).

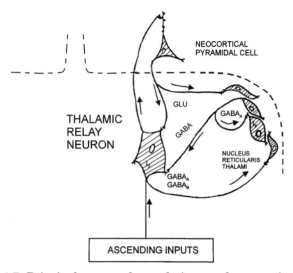

Fig. 1-7. Principal neuronal populations and connections of thalamocortical circuit generating absence seizures. IT, T-calcium current; GLU, glutamatergic transmission; GABA, GABAergic transmission. From ref. (8), with permission.

This circuit includes cortical pyramidal neurons, thalamic relay neurons, and the nucleus reticularis thalami (NRT). The principal synaptic connections of the thalamocortical circuit include glutamatergic fibers between neocortical pyramidal cells and the NRT, GABAergic fibers from NRT neurons that activate $GABA_A$ and $GABA_B$ receptors on thalamic relay neurons, and recurrent collateral GABAergic fibers from NRT neurons that activate $GABA_A$ receptors on adjacent NRT neurons. Thalamic relay neurons and the NRT are in a position to influence the flow of information between the thalamus and cerebral cortex.

Thalamic relay neurons and NRT neurones possess low threshold, transient Ca^{2+} channels (T-channels) which allow them to exhibit a burst-firing mode, followed by an inactive mode. Mild depolarization of these neurons is sufficient to activate these T-channels and to allow the influx of extracellular Ca^{2+}. Further depolarization produced by Ca^{2+} inflow will often exceed the threshold for firing a burst of action potentials. After T-channels are activated, they become inactivated rather quickly; hence, the name "transient." T-channels require a lengthy, intense hyperpolarization to remove their inactivation (a process termed "deinactivation"). The requisite hyperpolarization can be provided by $GABA_B$ receptors that are present on thalamic relay neurons. In animal models of absences, $GABA_B$ agonists produce an increase in seizure frequency (by facilitating deinactivation of T-channels) while $GABA_B$ antagonists reduce seizure frequency.

As noted previously, recurrent collateral GABAergic fibers from the NRT neurons activate $GABA_A$ receptors on adjacent NRT neurons. Activating $GABA_A$ receptors in the NRT, therefore, results in inhibition of GABAergic output to the thalamic relay neurons, and would serve to reduce hyperpolarization and delay deinactivation of the T-channels. In animal studies, injection of the $GABA_A$ agonists bilaterally into the NRT reduces absence-seizure frequency. However, $GABA_A$ activation of thalamic relay neurons would be expected to have the opposite effect, increasing depolarization and deinactivation of the T-channel.

The exact defect(s) in thalamocortical function, which causes absence seizures in humans, is uncertain. Animal models of absence seizure have shown both aberrations in the function of T-channel's function and an increase in $GABA_A$ receptors in comparison with controls.

C. Effects of Development

The basic mechanisms of epileptogenesis and propagation are different in the immature brain. The immature brain is more prone to seizures due to an imbalance between inhibition and excitation. In particular, there are age-related differences in response to GABA in different brain areas (see references for details).

REFERENCES

1. Annegers JF. Epidemiology of epilepsy. In: Wyllie E, (ed): *The treatment of epilepsy: principles and practice,* 2nd ed. Baltimore: Williams and Wilkins, 1997.

2. Ayala GF, Dichter M, Gummit RJ, Matsumoto H, Spencer WA. Genesis of epileptic interictal spikes: new knowledge of cortical feedback systems suggests a neurophysiologic explanation of brief paroxysms. *Brain Res* 1973;52:1–17.

3. Commission on Classification and Terminology of the International League Against Epilepsy. Proposal for revised clinical and electrocephalographic classification of epileptic seizures. *Epilepsia* 1981;22:489–501.

4. Commission on Classification and Terminology of the International League Against Epilepsy. Proposal for revised classification of epilepsies and epileptic syndromes. *Epilepsia* 1989;30:389–399.

5. Engel J, Dichter MA, Schwartzkroin PA. Basic mechanisms of human epilepsy. In: Engel J, Pedley TA, eds. *Epilepsy: a comprehensive textbook*. Philadelphia: Lippincott–Raven Publishers, 1997.

6. Engel J, Pedley TA, eds. *Epilepsy: a comprehensive textbook*. Philadelphia: Lippincott–Raven Publishers, 1997, Chaps. 1–11, 21–42, 67–69.

7. Hauser WA, Hesdorffer DC. *Epilepsy: frequency, causes and consequences*. New York: Demos, 1990.

8. Holmes GL. Basic mechanisms in epilepsy. *Intern Pediat* 1996;11:343–350.

9. Holmes GL. Epilepsy in the developing brain: lessons from the laboratory and clinic. *Epilepsia* 1997;38:12–30.

10. Hubbard JI, Llinas R, Quastel DMJ. *Electrophysiological analysis of synaptic transmission*. Philadelphia: Williams & Wilkins, 1969.

11. Jackson JH. Lectures of the diagnosis of epilepsy. In: Taylor J, ed. *Selected Writings of John H. Jackson*, vol. 1, New York: Basic Books, 1951.

12. Lothman EW. Pathphysiololgy of seizures and epilepsy in the mature and immature brain: cells, synapses, and circuits. In: Dodson WE, Pellock JM, eds. *Pediatric epilepsy diagnosis and therapy*. New York: Demos, 1993:1–15.

13. McNamara JO, Wader JA. Kindling model. In: Engel J, Pedley TA, eds. *Epilepsy: a comprehensive textbook*. Philadelphia: Lippincott–Raven Publishers, 1997.

14. Olsen RW, Avoli M. GABA and epileptogenesis. *Epilepsia* 1997;38:399–407.

15. Prince DA. Physiological mechanisms of focal epileptogensis. *Epilepsia* 1985;26(Suppl 1):S3–S14.

16. Steriade M, Llinas RR. The functional states of the thalamus and the associated neuronal interplay. *Physiol Rev* 1988;68:649–742.

17. Sutula TP. The pathology of the epilepsies: insights into the causes and consequences of epileptic syndromes. In: Dodson WE, Pollack JM, eds. *Pediatric epilepsy: diagnosis and therapy*. New York: Demos, 1993:37–44.

18. Wyllie E, ed. The treatment of epilepsy: principles and practice, 2nd ed. Baltimore: Williams and Wilkins, 1997, Chaps 2,4,5,8,10–12,21, and 22.

TYPES OF SEIZURES

Table 2-1. *International classification of epileptic seizures*

I.   Partial (Focal, Local) Seizures
  A. Simple Partial Seizures (Consciousness Not Impaired)
    1. With Motor Signs
    2. With Sensory Symptoms
    3. With Autonomic Symptoms or Signs
    4. With Psychic Symptoms
  B. Complex Partial Seizures (Temporal Lobe or Psychomotor Seizures; Consciousness Impaired)
    1. Simple Partial Onset, Followed by Impairment of Consciousness
      a. With Simple Partial Features (A1-A4), Followed by Impaired Consciousness
      b. With Automatisms
    2. With Impairment of Consciousness at Onset
      a. With Impairment of Consciousness Only
      b. With Automatisms
  C. Partial Seizures Evolving to Secondarily Generalized Seizures (Tonic-Clonic, Tonic or Clonic)
    1. Simple Partial Seizures (A) Evolving to Generalized Seizures
    2. Complex Partial Seizures (B) Evolving to Generalized Seizures
    3. Simple Partial Seizures Evolving to Complex Partial Seizures, Evolving to Generalized Seizures
II. Generalized Seizures (Convulsive or Nonconvulsive)
  A. Absence (Petit Mal) Seizures
  B. Myoclonic Seizures
  C. Tonic Seizures
  D. Atonic Seizures
  E. Clonic Seizures
  F. Tonic-Clonic (Grand Mal) Seizures
III. Unclassified Epileptic Seizures (Caused by Incomplete Data)

Modified from ref. (2), with permission.

Classifications of epileptic seizures are concerned with classifying each individual seizure as a single event based upon clinical and electroencephalogram (EEG) information. The classification of epileptic seizures used throughout this book is the most recent revision (1981) of the Clinical and Electroencephalographic Classification of Epileptic Seizures of the International League Against Epilepsy ("International Classification of Epileptic Seizures").

Visual illusions (distortions of visual input) and hallucinations (perception of a stimulus not actually present) usually represent seizure phenomena arising from the posterior temporal area.

Auditory seizures arising near the cortex of Heschel's region of the first temporal gyrus, may produce simple auditory phenomena usually described as a "humming," "buzzing," or "hissing." More complex auditory illusions or hallucinations result from discharges arising in the auditory association areas of the temporal lobe.

Olfactory and gustatory seizures consist of olfactory and gustatory illusions or hallucinations, usually in the form of unpleasant odors and tastes.

Vertiginous seizures may consist only of a vague feeling of dizziness or lightheadedness. Vertiginous sensations without alteration of consciousness are extremely frequent expressions of vestibular irritative phenomena (peripheral or central), although they have been described also as true epileptic manifestations of seizure foci in the middle or posterior portion of the first temporal gyrus (*"tornado epilepsy"*).

C. SIMPLE PARTIAL SEIZURES WITH AUTONOMIC SYMPTOMS OR SIGNS. These seizures may consist of epigastric sensations, flushing or pallor, sweating, pupillary dilatation, diaphoresis, piloerection, nausea, vomiting, borborygmi, or incontinence.

D. SIMPLE PARTIAL SEIZURES WITH PSYCHIC SYMPTOMS. Psychic symptoms may include: (a) dysphasia; (b) dysmnesia; (c) cognitive symptoms; (d) affective symptoms; (e) illusions; or (f) structured hallucinations.

Dysphasic symptoms may take the form of speech arrest, vocalization, or *palilalia* (involuntary repetition of a syllable or phrase).

Dysmnesic symptoms, distortions of memory, may take the form of a temporal disorientation, a dreamy state, a flashback, a sensation as if an experience had occurred before (*déja vu*, if visual; *déja entendu*, if auditory), or a sensation as if a previously experienced sensation had not been experienced (*jamais vu*, if visual; *jamais entendu*, if auditory). Occasionally, a patient may experience a rapid recollection of episodes from the past (panoramic vision).

Cognitive symptoms may include dreamy states, distortions of time sense, and sensations of unreality, detachment, or depersonalization.

Affective symptoms may include fear, pleasure, displeasure, depression, rage, anger, irritability, elation, and eroticism. Some individuals may have inappropriate affective reactions to environmental stimuli, possibly because of misinterpretation of cues during the clouded consciousness of a seizure. Fear is the most frequent affective symptom and may be accompanied by objective signs of autonomic activity such as pupil dilation, pallor, flushing, piloerection, palpitation, and hypertension.

Unlike the affective symptoms of psychiatric disease, those of partial seizures occur in attacks lasting a few minutes, tend to be unprovoked by environmental stimuli, and usually abate rapidly. Less commonly, patients describe exhilaration, elation, serenity, satisfaction, and pleasure (*ecstatic seizures, Dostoyevsky epilepsy*). The enjoyable sensations may be similar to or different from sexual pleasure. Sexual pleasure during an aura may consist of either sexual arousal or orgasm. *Violent affect* and behavior during partial seizures are discussed further on. *Illusions* are distorted perceptions in which objects are perceived as deformed. *Polyopic illusions* such as monocular diplopia, macropsia, micropsia, or distortions of distance may occur. Distortions of sound, including *microacusia* and *macroacusia*, may be experienced. *Depersonalization*, a feeling that the person is outside the body, may occur. The patient may experience altered perception of the size or weight of a limb.

Structural hallucinations are perceptions without corresponding external stimuli and may affect somatosensory, visual, auditory, olfactory, or gustatory senses. Seizures arising from primary receptive areas tend to give rather primitive hallucinations, whereas seizures arising from association areas tend to give more elaborate symptoms.

E. COMPLEX PARTIAL SEIZURES WITH SIMPLE PARTIAL ONSET. If a simple partial seizure arising in a circumscribed portion of one lobe spreads to involve larger portions of the brain and if consciousness becomes impaired, the seizure is classified in the group of "complex partial seizures with simple partial onset."

F. SIMPLE PARTIAL SEIZURES EVOLVING TO SECONDARILY GENERALIZED SEIZURES. Simple partial onset seizures may spread further and become secondarily generalized (tonic-clonic, tonic, or clonic).

3. EEG Phenomena

A. INTERICTAL EEG. Abnormal interictal EEGs are found in up to 80% to 90% of patients with simple partial seizures if multiple EEGs (including long-term monitoring) are performed and all types of abnormalities are considered. Only 50% or less of individual routine interictal EEGs show an abnormality. Focal spike or sharp discharges, slowing, or suppression of normal background are the usual abnormalities. There is an absence of focal EEG findings in many patients for several reasons: (a) spikes are an intermittent phenomenon; (b) spikes or slow waves originating from small areas of cortex may be markedly attenuated at the scalp; and (c) spikes or slow waves may originate from cortical areas distant from the convexity and be unrecorded at the scalp. Additional routine recordings, sleep deprivation, and long-term EEG recording increase the yield of abnormal EEG findings in a patient with a normal initial EEG.

B. ICTAL EEG. At the time of onset of clinical seizures, a majority of patients with focal seizures show a transformation in the scalp EEG from an interictal pattern to a sustained rhythmic pattern. The initial frequency of rhythmic ictal transformation (RIT) is most often in the range of 13 to 30 Hz but may be slower. The RIT shows a progressive increase in amplitude and a decrease in frequency as clinical seizures develop. Spread to adjacent areas of brain is indicated by the development of RIT in those areas. Termination of rhythmic ictal activity may be associated with the gradual development of slow-wave and spike-slow-wave activity that gradually decreases in frequency and then gives way to postictal slowing or depression of voltage, or both. Rhythmic ictal activity can also subside abruptly. In the minority of cases that show no RIT, the interictal pattern of mixed sharp and slow activity (or normal background) persists without observable change during the clinical seizure.

4. Basic Mechanisms
   See Chapter 1.

5. Differential Diagnosis
   Simple partial seizures in adults must be differentiated from migraine, syncope, transient ischemic attacks, Meniere's disease, and psychogenic seizures. In children, tics, chorea, and tremor sometimes cause diagnostic confusion. These differential diagnoses are discussed in Chapter 9.

*6. Epilepsy Types, Epilepsy Syndromes,
and Cerebral Localization*

Simple partial seizures usually occur as part of "localization-related/symptomatic epilepsy." Within this epilepsy there are four epilepsy syndromes named for the presumed location of onset: temporal lobe, frontal lobe, parietal lobe, or occipital lobe. See Chapter 1 for definitions and Chapter 3 for details.

7. Etiology, Management, Prognosis

These topics are reviewed in Chapter 3.

B. Complex Partial Seizures (Psychomotor or Temporal Lobe Seizures)

1. Definitions

The central feature of complex partial seizures (CPS) is *impairment of consciousness*. Impairment of consciousness is defined as the inability to respond normally to exogenous stimuli by virtue of altered awareness or responsiveness. Responsiveness refers to the ability of the patient to carry out simple commands or willed movement, and awareness refers to the patient's contact with events during the period in question and its recall.

The period of impairment of consciousness may or may not be preceded by symptoms or signs of a simple partial seizure. There may be no other manifestations during the period of impaired consciousness, or there may be *automatisms* (that is, nonreflex actions performed "automatically," without conscious volition and for which the patient has no recollection).

2. Seizure Phenomena

A. CLASSIFICATION. The International Classification of Epileptic Seizures divides CPS into four groups (Table 2-1): (1) CPS with simple partial onset followed by impairment of consciousness only; (2) CPS with simple partial onset followed by impaired consciousness and automatisms; (3) CPS with impairment of consciousness at onset with impairment of consciousness only; and (4) CPS with impairment of consciousness at onset with automatisms. Three major areas describe seizure phenomena during CPS: (1) impairment of consciousness; (2) types of simple partial onset; and (3) automatisms.

B. IMPAIRMENT OF CONSCIOUSNESS. Impairment of consciousness is defined previously. During the period of impaired consciousness a patient may look "vacant" or "frightened." Although sometimes able to recount vague sensations, the patients do not realize that anything more has occurred.

C. TYPES OF SIMPLE PARTIAL ONSET. Simple partial onset with motor signs, with somatosensory or special sensory symptoms, with autonomic symptoms or signs and with psychic symptoms are discussed previously. Psychic symptoms can occur without impairment of consciousness as part of a simple partial seizure. More commonly, psychic symptoms occur in association with impaired consciousness as part of a CPS. The frequent association of psychic symptoms and motor automatisms with CPS is responsible for the former term "psychomotor seizure."

D. AUTOMATISMS. An automatism is a more-or-less coordinated, involuntary motor activity occurring during the state of clouding of consciousness either in the course of, or after, an epileptic seizure, usually followed by amnesia of the event. The automatism may be simply a continuation of an activity that was going on when the seizure occurred, or it may be a new activity developed in association with the ictal impairment of consciousness. Usually the activity is commonplace in nature, often provoked by the subject's environment or by sensations during the seizure; fragmentary, primitive, infantile, or antisocial behavior is occasionally seen. Automatisms can be detected in more than 90% of CPS recorded on videotape.

Five types of phenomena may occur during an automatism: alimentary, mimetic, gestural, ambulatory, and verbal. *Alimentary* phenomena include: automatic chewing movements, increased salivation, or borborygmus. *Mimetic* phenomena include: movements of the face resulting in expressions of fear, bewilderment, discomfort, vacant tranquility, laughing (*gelastic seizures*), or crying (*lacrimonic seizures*). *Gestural* phenomena include: repetitive movements of the hands and fingers and sexual gestures. *Ambulatory* phenomena include wandering or running (*cursive seizures*), and the patient may unknowingly run out into traffic or into obstacles. *Verbal* phenomena include: short phrases, expletives, or swearing, commonly repeated in an automatic fashion. The spontaneous vocalization words may reflect a previous experience.

E. DROP ATTACKS. Sudden loss of consciousness, accompanied by loss of postural tone and falls may occur during a CPS. Such patients usually have had seizures for several years before the falls begin, suggesting an increasing rate of spread.

F. COMPOUND FORMS OF CPS. Most CPS exhibit a combination of the symptoms previously listed. Delgado-Escueta et al. (4) found that most CPS were compound forms of two types.

During the early phase of a *Type I* attack, the patient was essentially motionless and initially unresponsive to superficial and deep pain. After approximately 10 sec, a second phase of 10 to 60 sec duration was observed. During this time the patient remained unresponsive and showed automatisms such as repeated chewing, blinking, and swallowing. During the later third, the longest phase of type I (0.5 to 12 min), impairment of consciousness of a less profound nature was observed. Automatisms could be interrupted, and the patient sometimes reacted to environmental cues. This phase is best described as a "cloudy state."

Type II attacks consisted of reactive automatisms during impaired consciousness. A motionless, staring state was not observed, although stereotyped movements occurred. Automatisms occurring during the cloudy states of type II attacks and during the third phase of type I, attacks were considered reactive because the behavior appeared purposeful. Amnesia for the entire attack ensued. Motor responses were coordinated and were sufficient to carry out the patient's intended actions; they appeared both appropriate and inappropriate.

G. CPS EVOLVING TO GENERALIZED SEIZURES. The seizure discharges of a CPS may become secondarily generalized, producing a generalized seizure (tonic-clonic, tonic or clonic; see following).

H. CPS STATUS EPILEPTICUS. See Chapter 12.

3. EEG Phenomena

A. INTERICTAL. Interictal manifestations of CPS include focal spikes, sharp waves, and slowing. These abnormalities most often are found in the anterior temporal region, but many occur in other areas. Abnormalities may be localized or bilateral (synchronous or asynchronous). Discharges arising from the mesial surface of the frontal lobe may appear as generalized discharges on surface EEG.

B. ICTAL EEG. During a clinical CPS, any of the following can be recorded from scalp EEG electrodes: (a) sustained rhythm of spikes or sharp waves and rhythmic slowing; (b) attenuation of amplitude (suppression); (c) rhythmic slow waves; (d) 10- to 30-Hz fast activity; (e) spike-wave complexes; (f) other changes or variants of (a) to (e); or (g) no change (10% to 30% of patients). These patterns may be focal, lateralized, bilateral, or diffuse.

C. POSTICTAL EEG. The postictal EEG usually consists of generalized or localized slow activity. Localized postictal slowing provides information about lateralization or localization of the site of origin of the CPS in approximately 40% of recordings.

D. SPECIAL EEG TECHNIQUES. Approximately 50% of routine EEGs performed on patients with CPS are abnormal. This yield can be increased to 90% using repeated studies, sleep deprivation (allowing only 4 hr or less sleep the night before study), additional temporal electrodes (usually T1 and T2, alternatively sphenoidal electrodes), and long-term EEG monitoring. When CPS are suspected clinically and a routine EEG is normal, a sleep-deprived EEG with temporal leads should be ordered. If this is normal, long-term EEG monitoring should be considered.

4. Neurobehavioral Aspects of CPS

Patients with CPS often have: (a) damage to limbic structures (with resulting cognitive and behavioral problems); (b) seizures involving limbic structures; and (c) psychosocial difficulties caused by (a) and (b). Thus, there are a number of complex neurobehavioral issues associated with CPS.

A. EMOTIONAL ACTIVATION OF CPS. Patients with CPS are vulnerable to emotional activation of seizure activity because the anatomic structures involved during CPS are those that subserve normal emotional responses. Conversely, reducing emotional stress (which may happen during hospitalization) may decrease the occurrence of CPS.

B. INTERICTAL PERSONALITY. Several authors have described "an interictal personality" of patients with CPS, characterized by such features as "stickiness," humorlessness, dependence, obsessionalism, circumstantiality, philosophic interests, religiosity, anger, personalized significance attached to trivial events, hypergraphia, altered sexual interest (hyposexuality or hypersexuality), and emotionality.

Some patients with CPS do exhibit these traits. More studies are needed, however, to determine the prevalence of these traits in nonselected patients, their specificity for CPS, and the pathophysiology and psychodynamics of the trait. Pharmacologic or surgical control of seizures does not alter these personality traits.

C. VIOLENT BEHAVIOR. Attempts to restrain a patient who has clouded sensorium during or after a tonic-clonic or complex partial seizure may result in defensive and aggressive behavior. Well-organized, unprovoked, directed acts of violence are rarely a manifestation of epilepsy, however. Episodic dyscontrol syndrome (rage attacks) is not a form of CPS (see Chapter 9).

D. MEMORY LOSS. Poor memory and memory loss are frequent complaints of the patient with CPS. Short-term memory loss and subjective difficulty with memory have been attributed to hippocampal dysfunction in temporal lobe epilepsy. A major abnormality found on formal psychometric testing is poor performance on confrontation-naming tests in patients with CPS and a left-temporal EEG focus. This anomia, in turn, may result in impairment on many verbal subtests of intelligence and memory.

E. PSYCHOSIS. A psychosis resembling paranoid schizophrenia has been noted in some patients with CPS. Some have reported, and some have denied, that the psychosis of CPS can be differentiated from schizophrenia because patients with CPS retain more affect and are less socially isolated than are patients with schizophrenia.

F. EPISODES OF AIMLESS WANDERING (PORIOMANIA). Patients with CPS may experience prolonged episodes of aimless wandering followed by retrograde amnesia for this behavior. This may represent a prolonged postictal automatism and has been reported to respond to antiepileptic medication.

5. Basic Mechanisms
See Chapter 1.

6. Differential Diagnosis
In adults, complex partial seizures must be differentiated from absence seizures, syncope, transient ischemic attacks, episodic dyscontrol syndrome, psychosis, Meniere's disease, and psychogenic seizures. In children, night terrors and sleep walking must also be considered. These differential diagnoses are discussed in Chapter 9.

*7. Epilepsy Types, Epilepsy Syndromes, and
Cerebral Localization*
Complex partial seizures usually occur as part of "localization-related/symptomatic epilepsy." Within this epilepsy there are four epilepsy syndromes named for the presumed location of onset: temporal lobe, frontal lobe,

parietal lobe, or occipital lobe. See Chapter 1 for definitions and Chapter 3 for details.

8. Etiology, Management, Prognosis
These topics are reviewed in Chapter 3.

C. Partial Seizures Evolving to Secondarily Generalized (Tonic-Clonic, Grand Mal) Seizures

1. Definitions
Tonic-clonic seizures consist of an initial increase in
tone of certain muscles (tonic phase) followed by bilateral symmetrical jerking of the extremities (clonic phase).

Secondarily generalized tonic-clonic seizures begin
with focal seizure activity and may be accompanied by
clinical or EEG evidence of simple and/or complex partial
seizures.

Tonic-clonic seizures most often occur as part of local-
ization-related/symptomatic (partial, focal) epilepsy.
However, tonic-clonic seizures may occur as part of many
other adult epilepsy syndromes (see Tables 3-1, 4-1, 5-1,
6-1, 7-1, 8-1). Regardless of epilepsy syndrome, tonic-
clonic seizures share a number of common features presented in this section. Special features of tonic-clonic
seizures associated with localization-related/sympto-
matic (partial, focal) epilepsy also are reviewed in this
section. Special features of tonic-clonic seizures associated with other specific epilepsy syndromes are reviewed
with the specific epilepsy syndrome in Chapters 3–8.

2. Seizure Phenomena (Fig. 2-1)
A. AURA. Secondarily generalized tonic-clonic seizures
may begin with signs or symptoms of focal seizure phenomena appropriate to the focus of origin (simple partial
and/or complex partial seizure phenomena, see aforemen-
tioned). However, most patients cannot recall an aura.
B. TONIC PHASE. The tonic phase usually consists of a
brief phase in flexion, followed by a longer phase in extension. Consciousness is lost during the tonic phase. The
flexion phase usually begins in the face (eyes open, ocular
globes rotated upward, mouth held rigidly open), neck
(held rigid in semiflexion), and trunk (chest bent forward
on pelvis). The flexion phase then spreads to the extremities, involving the arms more than the legs and the proximal muscles more than the distal muscles. The arms are
elevated, adducted, and externally rotated, and the legs
and thighs are flexed, adducted, and externally rotated.

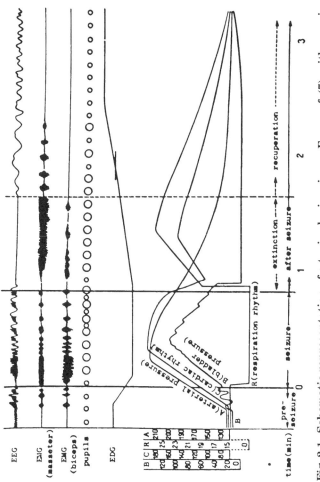
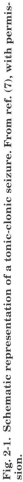

Fig. 2-1. Schematic representation of a tonic-clonic seizure. From ref. (7), with permission.

The *extension phase* begins in the axial musculature with extension of the back and neck. The mouth snaps shut (the tongue may be bitten). The thoracic and abdominal muscles then contract, sometimes producing a "tonic cry" as air is forced over the vocal cords. The arms are lowered and adducted. The forearm may remain flexed or may be extended and pronated. Fingers may be clenched upon the extended wrists or extended upon flexed wrists. The legs are extended, adducted, and externally rotated.

During the period of transition from the tonic to the clonic phase (*"vibratory tonic period"*), tetanus becomes less complete. Tonic rigidity is replaced by a fine tremor, which increases in amplitude and decreases in frequency from 8 to 4 Hz. The tremor is caused by intermittent decreases in tone. The tremor begins in the extremities and spreads proximally.

C. CLONIC PHASE. During the clonic phase, muscle relaxation completely interrupts tonic contraction. The rhythmic return of muscle tone causes the appearance of rhythmic jerks, which become farther and farther apart until the seizure ends. The tongue may be bitten owing to clonic masseter movements. Each jerk may be accompanied by a cry.

D. AUTONOMIC PHENOMENA. Autonomic phenomena begin in the preictal phase, are maximal at the end of the tonic phase, and decrease abruptly at the onset of the clonic phase. Autonomic phenomena that may be observed during a tonic-clonic seizure include: increased blood pressure, increased heart rate, increased bladder pressure, increased sphincter tone, flushing, cyanosis, piloerection, perspiration, increased salivation, and increased bronchial secretion.

Apnea begins with violent expiration at the onset of the tonic phase and persists during the tonic and clonic phases (except for violent, forced expirations with clonic jerks), and often into the early postictal period. Apnea cannot be explained entirely on the basis of muscular contractions; a central mechanism is probably involved in maintaining it.

E. IMMEDIATE POSTICTAL PHASE. Complete muscular relaxation does not occur immediately. About 5 sec after the last clonic jerk, there is a new period of tonic contraction lasting from several sec to 4 min. Muscle tone is most increased in the cephalic muscles, and the tongue may be bitten. The trunk and arms may be extended but not as violently as during the tonic phase.

Between the last clonic jerk and the immediate postictal tonic phase, the bladder sphincter muscles relax; at this point incontinence may occur.

Respirations return during the immediate postictal phase. The combination of a clenched jaw and increased secretions results in partial obstruction of respiration. Respirations are stertorous, and accessory muscles of respiration are activated. Blood pressure and skin resistance return to normal, but tachycardia persists. Cyanosis changes to pallor. Loss of consciousness remains complete, and pupillary and cutaneous reflexes are absent. Deep tendon reflexes are variably modified.

F. LATER POSTICTAL PHASE. In this phase there is, more or less, complete flaccidity. The cardiac rate returns to normal. Deep tendon reflexes are usually diminished, and the plantar response is sometimes extensor. The patient may awaken by passing through successive stages of coma, confusional state, and drowsiness or may pass directly into sleep without awakening.

G. DURATION OF PHASES. The average duration of the various phases of a tonic-clonic seizure are as follows: tonic phase, 10 to 30 sec; clonic phase, 30 to 50 sec; immediate postictal phase, 1 to 5 min; later postictal phase, 2 to 10 min; total, 5 to 15 min. Individual phase duration and clinical expression are highly variable in partial seizures secondarily generalized, suggesting multiple routes of spread.

H. TONIC-CLONIC STATUS EPILEPTICUS. See Chapter 12.

3. Complications

The possible complications of tonic-clonic seizures, in order of likelihood, are summarized in the following. Tonic-clonic status epilepticus increases the risk of all these complications.

Oral Trauma: The tongue, lip, or check may be macerated. *Head Trauma:* Skull fractures, contusions, and epidural or subdural hematomas may result from head injury caused by falls or clonic activity. *Stress Fractures:* Compression fractures of thoracic or lumbar vertebrae may occur; they are often asymptomatic and more common in the elderly. *Aspiration Pneumonia:* Aspiration of secretions or regurgitated stomach contents may occur when the airway's normal protective reflexes are inhibited postictally, and may be life-threatening. *Postictal Pulmonary Edema:* This is a rare complication (immediate or delayed) manifested by dyspnea, cough, blood-stained sputum, and abnormal chest x-ray. This complication usually requires only oxygen therapy and needs to be differentiated from aspiration pneumonia.

4. EEG Phenomena (Fig. 2-1)

A. **INTERICTAL PHASE.** Focal spikes, sharp waves, or slowing may be present (see simple partial seizures and complex partial seizures previously).

B. **PREICTAL PHASE.** During the preictal phase of a secondarily generalized tonic-clonic seizure, the EEG may show focal attenuation, sharp waves, or slow activity.

C. **TONIC PHASE.** The tonic phase begins with a 1- to 3-sec period of EEG flattening ("desynchronization") or with low-voltage fast activity. Then, surface negative waves at about 10 Hz appear and increase rapidly in amplitude ("epileptic recruiting rhythm"). After approximately 10 sec, the recruiting rhythm becomes combined with an apparently separate rhythm of slow waves, increasing in amplitude and decreasing in frequency from 3 to 1 Hz. The slow rhythm becomes progressively more prominent and the recruiting rhythm becomes progressively less prominent until the recruiting rhythm appears only as brief bursts of rapid activity between surface-negative slow waves.

D. **CLONIC PHASE.** During the clonic phase bursts of 10 Hz recruiting rhythm alternate with slow waves. Bursts of recruiting rhythm are associated with generalized jerks, and slow waves are associated with relaxation. The slow waves become slower and the bursts of recruiting rhythm become farther apart.

E. **POSTICTAL PHASE.** The EEG is isoelectric for a few sec to 1 min after the last clonic jerk ("cortical exhaustion"). Then, low-voltage, very slow activity appears. The EEG then progressively picks up in voltage and frequency.

5. Basic Mechanisms
See Chapter 1.

6. Differential Diagnosis
Partial seizures evolving to secondarily generalized seizures, occurring as part of localization related/symptomatic epilepsies, must be differentiated from primarily generalized tonic-clonic seizures occurring as part of generalized/idiopathic epilepsies (see Tables 1-2, 5-1, 6-1, 7-1, 8-1). Secondarily generalized seizures are suggested by: (a) evidence of structural brain damage (neurologic examination, imaging studies); (b) onset with symptoms or

signs suggesting simple and/or complex partial seizure; and (c) focal sharp or slow activity on interictal EEG. Primarily generalized seizures are suggested by: (a) absence of evidence of structural brain damage; (b) positive family history for seizures; (c) co-existing myoclonic or absence seizures; (d) occurrence shortly after awakening; (e) aura of bilateral myoclonic jerks; and (f) generalized spike-wave or polyspike wave on icterictal EEG.

Tonic-clonic seizures must also be distinguished from syncope and psychogenic seizures in patients of all ages. In children, tonic-clonic seizures must be distinguished from breath-holding spells and prolonged QT syndrome. These differential diagnoses are discussed in Chapter 9.

7. Epilepsy Types, Epilepsy Syndromes, and Cerebral Localization

Partial seizures secondarily generalized usually occur as part of "localization-related/symptomatic epilepsy." Within this epilepsy there are four epilepsy syndromes named for the presumed location of onset: temporal lobe, frontal lobe, parietal lobe, or occipital lobe. See Chapter 1 for definitions and Chapter 3 for details.

8. Etiology, Management, Prognosis

These topics are reviewed in Chapter 3.

II. GENERALIZED SEIZURES (CONVULSIVE OR NONCONVULSIVE)

A. Absence (Petit Mal) Seizures

1. Definitions

Absence seizures are generalized seizures, indicating bihemispheric, initial involvement clinically and electroencephalographically. They have a rapid onset and offset and most frequently are characterized by a change in facial expression, motionless blank staring, and with longer seizures, automatisms. Absence seizures are divided into typical and atypical (Table 2-2). As will be discussed, many children with absence seizures can be further categorized as having a characteristic epileptic syndrome.

2. Seizure Phenomena

A. TYPICAL ABSENCE SEIZURES. Although typical absence seizures may occur at any age, they rarely start before the age of 2 or after the teenage years. The hallmark of the typical absence is the suppression of mental function,

Table 2-2. *Classification of absence seizures*

I. Typical absence seizures
  A. Simple—impairment of consciousness only
  B. Complex
     a. With mild clonic components
     b. With changes in tone
     c. With automatisms
     d. With autonomic components
II. Atypical absence seizures
III. Absence status epilepticus

usually to the point of complete abolition of awareness, responsiveness, and memory. The seizures start abruptly, without an aura, and typically last from a few seconds to half a minute, although, at times, they last over a minute. Ongoing activity is suddenly interrupted; the child changes facial expression and becomes transfixed (like a statue). In a *simple typical absence seizure*, the child stares with a motionless, distant appearance. At the end of the seizure the child usually returns to the gesture, sentence, or other activity that the seizure interrupted. Postictal fatigue never occurs, although the child may be momentarily confused caused by the "time loss." This "time loss" may serve as a clue to the child that a seizure occurred, even though there may be complete amnesia for events during the seizure.

Maximum impairment of responsiveness usually occurs during the first few seconds of an absence seizure, regardless of whether the total duration of the seizure is brief or long. At times, the suspension of mental function is less complete, especially at the end of certain longer attacks. At this time, there may be mild confusion without complete loss of awareness. When this happens, the child may be able to continue simple and automatic behavior. At times, the impairment of consciousness is so slight that it passes unnoticed by observers and may be detected only during EEG monitoring.

Simple absence seizures are relatively rare. The majority of typical absence seizures are *complex typical absence seizures*, consisting of clonic or myoclonic activity, automatisms, and changes in postural tone. Automatisms occur frequently in absence seizures. Automatic behavior may consist of licking the lips, chewing, grimacing, scratching, or fumbling with the clothes. The longer the seizure is, the more likely that automatisms will occur.

More complex activity, such as dealing cards, or moving chess pieces may occur if it is ongoing at the onset of the seizure. While speech may continue to occur during an absence seizure, the speed usually slows.

B. ATYPICAL ABSENCE SEIZURES. Atypical absences are those seizures in which the onset and/or cessation are not as abrupt as in typical absences, and where changes in tone are more pronounced than in typical absences. Atypical absences, like typical absences, may be associated with automatisms, clonic components, and autonomic components, as well as changes in tone. However, automatisms are not as frequently seen in atypical absences as in typical absences. Atypical absence seizures frequently have a longer duration than typical absences, sometimes lasting several minutes.

C. ABSENCE STATUS EPILEPTICUS. This topic is reviewed in Chapter 12.

3. EEG Phenomena

A hallmark of absence seizures is the sudden onset of either generalized symmetrical spike-wave or multiple spike-and-slow-wave complexes. In typical absence seizures, the spike-and-wave complexes usually occur at a frequency of 3 Hz (range: 2.5–3.5 Hz) (see Fig. 2-2). At times, the discharge may begin with frontal spikes, occurring either unilaterally or bilaterally. Only when the spikes are persistently focal and precede the generalized discharge by several seconds, should a partial seizure with secondary generalization be considered. Likewise, following a generalized discharge there may be a second or two of rhythmic frontal delta activity without spikes.

Hyperventilation is a potent activator of typical absence seizures. Failure to induce an absence seizure with several trials of hyperventilation of 3 to 5 min duration in an untreated patient would make the diagnosis of absence seizures unlikely. Photic stimulation may also induce absence seizures, although the frequency for activation is not as high as with hyperventilation.

Focal spikes, particularly in the frontal region, or bilateral frontal spike-and-wave discharges are commonly seen in children with absence seizures. It has been suggested that these represent remnants of generalized discharges that did not fully propagate to the surface of the brain.

Unlike the usual 3 Hz spike-and-wave discharges that occur in typical absence seizures, slow spike-and-wave discharges occurring at 1.5 to 2.5 Hz are more characteristic of atypical absence seizures (see Fig. 2-3). The inter-

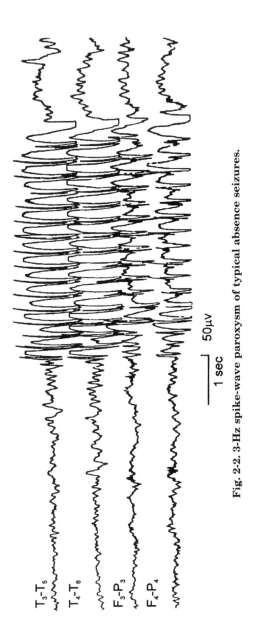

Fig. 2-2. 3-Hz spike-wave paroxysm of typical absence seizures.

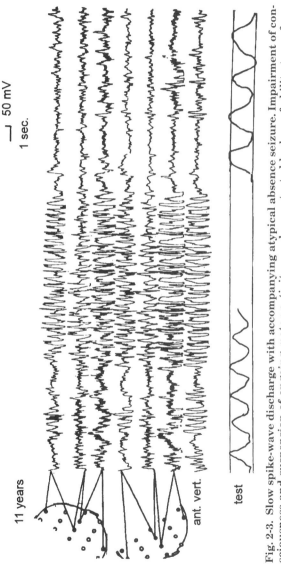

Fig. 2-3. Slow spike-wave discharge with accompanying atypical absence seizure. Impairment of consciousness and suspension of ongoing motor activity are demonstrated by loss of ability to perform simple writing task at bottom of the EEG paper. From ref.(8), with permission.

ictal EEG is usually abnormal in patients with atypical absences.

4. Basic Mechanisms

The pathophysiology of absence seizures is discussed in Chapter 1.

5. Differential Diagnosis

Absence seizures must be differentiated from complex partial seizures and daydreaming. The differential diagnosis of absence seizures from complex partial seizures is discussed in Chapter 9.

Daydreaming is associated with boredom, can be "broken" with stimulation, and is not associated with motor activity. Absence seizures, however, can sometimes be terminated with stimulation and tend to increase during periods of relaxation and tiredness. A normal EEG which includes several trials of 3 to 5 min of hyperventilation, however, virtually rules out absence seizures.

6. Epilepsy Types and Epilepsy Syndrome.

Typical absence seizures usually occur as part of generalized/idiopathic epilepsies and may be part of three epilepsy syndromes: childhood absence epilepsy syndrome, juvenile absence epilepsy syndrome, and juvenile myoclonic epilepsy syndrome (see Chapters 6 and 7). Atypical absence seizures occur as part of generalized/symptomatic epilepsies and the Lennox-Gastaut syndrome (see Chapter 6).

7. Etiology

The lack of structural pathology and the age-specific window observed in most patients with *typical absence seizures* implicate a hereditary etiology. Patients with *atypical absence seizures* have a higher likelihood of acquired disease. Often, patients with atypical absence seizures will have the Lennox-Gastaut syndrome which will be discussed in Chapter 6.

8. Management and Prognosis

See Chapters 6 and 7.

B. Myoclonic Seizures

1. Definition

Myoclonic seizures are characterized by sudden, brief (<350 msec), shocklike contractions that may be generalized or confined to the face and trunk, or to one or more extremities, or even to individual muscles or groups of muscles. Myoclonic seizures result in short bursts of synchronized electromyographic activity, which often involves simultaneous activation of agonist and antagonist muscles. The contractions of muscles are quicker than the contractions with clonic seizures.

2. Seizure Phenomena

Any group of muscles can be involved in a myoclonic seizure. Myoclonic seizures may be dramatic, causing the patient to fall to the ground, or be quite subtle, resembling tremors. Because of the brevity of the seizures, it is not possible to determine if consciousness is impaired.

While myoclonic seizures can sometimes be the only seizure type, myoclonic seizures often occur in combination with other seizure types.

3. EEG Phenomena

Myoclonic seizures are typically associated with generalized spike-and-wave or multiple spike-and-wave discharges on the EEG. In early myoclonic epileptic encephalopathy, the EEG demonstrates a burst-suppression pattern.

Myoclonic jerks may be correlated with bursts of generalized epileptiform discharges, but there may be no obvious link between the EEG discharges and myoclonic jerks recorded using EMG techniques, the so-called "EEG-EMG dissociation." However, back-averaging of EEG at the time of the EMG discharge may demonstrate a time link between the two events. Myoclonic seizures are frequently associated with exaggerated photosensitivity.

4. Differential Diagnosis

Myoclonic jerks are so brief that they may be missed by parents and physicians. Once seen, the diagnosis is usually not difficult. Like simple partial seizures, myoclonic seizures may occasionally be confused with tics.

5. Etiology

Myoclonic seizures can be seen in both acquired and familial disorders. Virtually any etiologic agent that leads to brain damage can be associated with myoclonic seizures. Therefore, myoclonic seizures are a part of many epilepsy types and many epilepsy syndromes (see below).

6. Epilepsy Types and Epilepsy Syndromes

Myoclonic seizures occur at all ages, from neonates to the elderly. Myoclonic seizures may be part of the following epilepsy types: generalized/idiopathic, generalized/symptomatic, generalized/either idiopathic or symptomatic, both localization-related and generalized, situation-related, and special syndromes. Myoclonic seizures may be part of a large number of epilepsy syndromes listed in Tables 3-1, 4-1, 5-1, 6-1, and 7-1.

7. Management and Prognosis
    See Chapters 3-7.

C and D. Tonic and Atonic Seizures

1. Definitions
    Tonic seizures are brief seizures consisting of the sudden onset of increased tone in the extensor muscles. If standing, the patient typically falls to the ground. Their duration is longer than myoclonic seizures. Electromyographic activity is dramatically increased in tonic seizures. Conversely, *atonic seizures* consist of the sudden loss of muscle tone. The loss of muscle tone may be confined to a group of muscles, such as the neck, resulting in a head drop, or involve all trunk muscles, leading to a fall to the ground.

2. Seizure Phenomena
    Tonic seizures frequently begin with a tonic contraction of the neck muscles, leading to fixation of the head in an erect position, widely opened eyes, and jaw-clenching or mouth-opening. Contraction of the respiratory and abdominal muscles often follows, and may lead to a high-pitched cry and brief periods of apnea. The tonic contractions may extend to the proximal musculature of the upper limbs, elevating the shoulders, and abducting the arms. Asymmetrical tonic seizures vary from a slight rotation of the head to a tonic contraction of all the musculature of one side of the body. Occasionally, tonic seizures terminate with a clonic phase. Eyelid retraction, staring, mydriasis, and apnea are commonly associated with the motor activity and may be the most prominent features. The seizures may cause falls and injury.
    Tonic seizures are typically activated by sleep and may occur repetitively throughout the night. They are much more frequent during non-REM sleep than during wakefulness and usually do not occur during REM sleep. During tonic seizures the patient is unconscious, although arousal from light sleep may occur. Since they are often very brief, they often go undetected. Tonic seizures are usually brief, lasting from a few seconds to a minute, with an average duration of about 10 sec. In seizures lasting

longer than a few seconds, impairment of consciousness is usually apparent. Postictal impairment with confusion, tiredness, and headache is common. The degree of postictal impairment is usually related to the duration of the seizure.

Atonic seizures begin suddenly and without warning and cause the patient, if standing, to fall quickly to the floor. Since there may be total lack of tone, the patient has no means to protect himself or herself. Injuries often occur. The attack may be fragmentary and lead to dropping of the head with slackening of the jaw or, dropping of a limb. In atonic seizures there should be a loss of electromyographic activity. Consciousness is impaired during the fall, although the patient may regain alertness immediately upon hitting the floor.

Tonic and atonic seizures can occur at all ages. However, they most often begin during childhood as part of one of several epilepsy syndromes listed below.

3. EEG Phenomena

The interictal EEG of patients with *tonic seizures* is usually quite abnormal, consisting of slowing of the background, with multifocal spikes, sharp waves, and bursts of irregular spike-and-wave activity. The EEG-ictal manifestations of tonic seizures usually consist of bilateral synchronous spikes of 10 to 25 Hz of medium-to-high voltage, with a frontal accentuation. Simple flattening or desynchronization may also occur. Occasionally, multiple spike-and-wave or diffuse, slow activity may occur during a tonic seizure.

Atonic seizures are usually associated with rhythmic spike-and-wave complexes varying from slow, 1 to 2 Hz, to more rapid, irregular spike- or multiple spike-and-wave activity.

4. Differential Diagnosis

Tonic seizures are usually not difficult to diagnose. Sometimes children with very severe encephalopathies have episodes of *opisthotonic posturing* that may resemble tonic seizures. Recording an episode usually helps distinguish the two events; tonic seizures would be associated with spike-wave discharges or a discharge of rapid spikes, while no epileptiform discharges should be seen during opisthotic posturing.

Paroxysmal choreoathetosis is a rare, usually familial, disorder characterized by episodic attacks of severe dystonia, choreoathetosis, or both. Two types have been described: paroxysmal dystonic choreoathetosis of Mount and Reback and paroxysmal kinesigenic choreoathetosis. In *paroxysmal dystonic choreoathetosis*, the patient has a sudden onset of severe, often painful, dystonia that may affect the arms, legs, or trunk and speech. Consciousness is not impaired during the attacks, which last from minutes to hours and are often precipitated by alcohol, caffeine, excitement, stress, or fatigue. The disorder is inherited through an autosomal-dominant pattern. *Paroxysmal kinesigenic choreoathetosis* is characterized by the sudden assumption of dystonic posturing or choreoathetosis. The kinesigenic attacks are usually shorter in duration than the dystonic form, and are frequently induced by sudden movements or a startle. These attacks can occur hundreds of times daily.

Spasmus nutans is a disorder occurring in toddlers which is characterized by head tilt, head nodding, and nystagmus, which is often asymmetric. The head nodding may be confused with atonic seizures. Spasms nutans is usually a self-limiting condition, disappearing after a period of 4 months to several years.

5. Etiology
Virtually any disorder that can lead to brain damage may result in tonic and atonic seizures. Common etiologies include hypoxic-ischemic encephalopathy, head injuries, encephalitis, strokes, congenital brain anomalies, and metabolic disturbances.

6. Epilepsy Types and Epilepsy Syndromes
Tonic and atonic seizures most often occur as part of generalized/symptomatic epilepsies and one of the following epilepsy syndromes: atonic seizures, tonic seizures, Lennox-Gastaut syndrome (see Chapter 6). Tonic seizures also may occur as part of neonatal seizures (see Chapter 4) or febrile convulsions (see Chapter 8). Atonic seizures also may occur as part of myoclonic-akinetic epilepsy syndrome (see Chapter 6).

7. Management and Prognosis
See Chapters 4, 6, and 8.

E. Clonic Seizures
Clonic seizures occur almost exclusively in neonates and young children. The attack begins with loss or impairment of consciousness, associated with sudden hypotonia or a brief, generalized tonic spasm. This is fol-

lowed by one to several minutes of bilateral jerks, which are often asymmetric and may predominate in one limb. During the attack there may be great variability in the amplitude, frequency, and spatial distribution of these jerks from moment to moment. In other children, particularly those aged 1 to 3 years, the jerks remain bilateral and synchronous throughout the attack. Postictally, there may be rapid recovery or a prolonged period of confusion or coma.

F. Tonic-Clonic (Grand Mal) Seizures

1. Definitions, Seizure Phenomena, EEG Phenomena, and Differential Diagnosis

The tonic-clonic seizures associated with generalized seizures are similar in most clinical and EEG respects to tonic-clonic seizures associated with partial seizures. The differences in these two seizure types are reviewed previously.

2. Epilepsy Types and Epilepsy Syndromes

Generalized-onset tonic-clonic seizures may occur as part of the following epilepsy types: generalized/idiopathic, generalized/symptomatic, generalized/either idiopathic or symptomatic, both localization-related and generalized, and special situations. The many epilepsy syndromes which may occur as part of these epilepsies are listed in Table 1-2.

3. Management and Prognosis

General management of tonic-clonic seizures is reviewed in Chapter 3. Prognosis of specific syndromes containing tonic-clonic seizures is reviewed in Chapters 3 , 5, 6, and 7.

REFERENCES

1. Browne TR, Feldman RG, eds. *Epilepsy: diagnosis and management*. Boston: Little Brown, 1983. (Contains series of reviews of seizure types.)
2. Commission on Classification and Terminology of the International League Against Epilepsy. Proposal for revised clinical and electroencephalographic classification of epileptic seizures. *Epilepsia* 1981;22:489–501.
3. Commission on Classification and Terminology of the International League Against Epilepsy. Proposal for revised classification of epilepsies and epileptic syndromes. *Epilepsia* 1989;30:389–399.

4. Delgado-Escueta AV, Bascal FE, Treiman D. Complex partial seizures on closed-circuit television and EEG: a study of 691 attacks on 79 patients. *Ann Neurol* 1982;11:292–300.

5. Engel J, Pedley TA, eds. *Epilepsy: a comprehensive textbook.* Philadelphia: Lippincott–Raven, 1997, Chaps. 43–58.

6. Gambardella A, Reutens DC, Anderman F, et al. Late onset drop attacks in temporal lobe epilepsy. *Neurology* 1994;44:1074–1078.

7. Gastaut H. Generalized convulsive seizures without local onset. In: Vinken PJ, Bruyn GW, eds. *Handbook of clinical neurology, Vol 15, The epilepsies.* Amsterdam: Elsevier, 1974.

8. Gastaut H. Generalized nonconvulsive seizures without local onset. In: Vinken PJ, Bruyn GW, eds. *Handbook of clinical neurology, Vol 15, The epilepsies.* Amsterdam: Elsevier, 1974.

9. Holmes GL. Myoclonic, tonic, and atonic seizures in children. *J Epilepsy* 1988;1:173–195.

10. Pearl PL, Holmes GL. Absence seizures. In: Dodson WE, Pellock JM, eds. *Pediatric epilepsy: diagnosis and therapy.* New York: Demos, 1993.

11. Penry JK, Porter RJ, Dreifuss FE. Simultaneous recording of absence seizures with videotape and electroencephalography. A study of 374 seizures in 48 patients. *Brain* 1975;98:427–447.

12. Theodore WH, Porter RJ, Albert P, et al. The secondarily generalized tonic-clinic seizure: a videotape analysis. *Neurology* 1994;44:1403–1407.

13. Wyllie E, ed. *The treatment of epilepsy: principles and practice*, 2nd ed. Baltimore: Williams and Wilkins, 1997, Chaps 21, 23–29.

3

EPILEPSIES WITH ONSET AT ALL AGES

TABLE 3-1. *Epilepsies and epilepsy syndromes with onset at all ages and accompanying seizure types*

I. Localization related/symptomatic (focal, partial) epilepsies
   A. Temporal lobe epilepsy syndromes (SPS, CPS, TCS)
   B. Frontal lobe epilepsy syndromes (SPS, CPS, TCS)
   C. Parietal lobe epilepsy syndromes (SPS, CPS, TCS)
   D. Occipital lobe epilepsy syndromes (SPS, CPS, TCS)
   E. Etiology
   F. Management
   G. Prognosis

SPS = simple partial (focal) seizures; CPS = complex partial (psychomotor, temporal lobe) seizures; TCS = tonic-clonic (grand mal) seizures.

There is one group of epilepsies with onset in patients of all ages: localization-related/symptomatic (focal, partial) epilepsies. These epilepsies are listed in Table 3-1, which forms an outline of this chapter.

Based upon seizure and EEG characteristics, age and evidence of brain pathology, a patient with localization-related/symptomatic epilepsy often can be classified into one of four groups of epilepsy syndromes, according to the presumed cerebral lobe in which seizures originate: temporal lobe, frontal lobe, parietal lobe, or occipital lobe (see Table 3-1). There is extensive and sometimes conflicting literature on cerebral localization using clinical and EEG data. Following is a summary of features agreed upon by the Commission on Classification and Terminology of the International League Against Epilepsy (6). For more detailed reviews, the reader is referred to references at the end of this chapter.

I. LOCALIZATION-RELATED/SYMPTOMATIC (PARTIAL, FOCAL) EPILEPSIES

A. Temporal Lobe Epilepsies

1. General Characteristics

Simple partial, complex partial, or secondarily generalized seizures (reviewed in Chapter 2) may occur. Onset is frequently in childhood or young adulthood. Seizures may occur randomly, at intervals, or in clusters. The simple partial seizures are characterized by autonomic and/or psychic symptoms and certain sensory phenomena such as olfactory and auditory illusions, or hallucinations. The most common sensation is a rising epigastric sensation.

2. Routine EEG Characteristics

Routine EEGs may show: (1) no abnormality; (2) slight or marked asymmetry of the background activity; or (3) temporal spikes, sharp waves, or slow waves (unilateral or bilateral, synchronous or asychronous, may not be confined to temporal areas).

3. Subtypes

A. AMYGDALA-HIPPOCAMPAL SEIZURES. These are the most common form of temporal lobe epilepsy and generally conform to the previous description. Seizures are characterized by rising epigastric discomfort, nausea, marked autonomic signs, and other symptoms including borborygmi, belching, pallor, fullness of the face, flushing, arrest of respiration, pupillary dilatation, fear, panic, and olfactory-gustatory hallucinations. The scalp EEG often shows unilateral or bilateral spikes most prominent in the anterior temporal leads.

One variant of amygdala-hippocampal seizures is the "mesial temporal lobe epilepsy syndrome." Such patients demonstrate mesial temporal sclerosis (defined later in this chapter) on imaging studies. Such patients typically have a strong family history of epilepsy and experience febrile seizures (often complicated) during infancy or childhood. After a silent period lasting 2 to 15 years, unprovoked partial seizures begin in late childhood or early adolescence. The seizures are refractory to medical treatment in 20% to 30% of patients. See French et al. (9) for details.

B. LATERAL TEMPORAL SEIZURES. These begin as simple partial seizures characterized by auditory hallucinations or illusions, dreamy state, visual misperceptions, or language disorders (dominant-hemisphere focus). These may progress to complex partial seizures if propagation to mesial temporal or extra temporal structures occurs. The scalp EEG often shows unilateral or bilateral spikes most prominent in the middle or posterior temporal leads.

B. Frontal Lobe Epilepsies

1. Clinical Characteristics

Frontal lobe epilepsies are characterized by simple partial, complex partial, or secondarily generalized seizures (reviewed in Chapter 2), or combinations of these. Features suggesting frontal lobe epilepsies are: (a) frequent seizures, often in sleep; (b) short seizure duration; (c) minimal or no postictal confusion after complex partial seizure; (d) rapid secondary generalization; (e) prominent motor manifestations which are tonic or postural; (f) complex gestural automatisms (may be sexual) at onset; (g) frequent falling during seizure; and (h) frequent episodes of status epilepticus.

2. EEG Characteristics

The interictal EEG may show: (a) no abnormality (especially if the focus is removed from the surface, e.g., orbitofrontal or supplementary motor area foci); (b) background asymmetry; and (c) spikes or sharp waves which can be unilateral or bilateral, unilobular or multilobular. Frontal seizure foci not infrequently exhibit spikes or sharp waves in temporal leads.

3. Subtypes

A. SUPPLEMENTARY MOTOR SEIZURES. These are typically brief, lasting only 10 to 40 sec. The patient develops abrupt tonic posturing of one or more extremities, the arms are affected more often than the legs. Characteristically, arms and legs are tonically adducted. During the tonic phase, the patient may cry or moan loudly. Consciousness is usually preserved, but the patient may be unable to speak. A versive movement, usually away from the side of ictal onset, may precede secondary generalization. The tonic posturing may be preceded by sensory symptoms in an extremity. Supplementary motor seizures occur frequently, and 5 to 10 episodes per day is not rare. Many occur during sleep. Commonly, these seizures are medically intractable.

B. CINGULATE. Cingulate seizure patterns are complex partial with complex motor gestural automatisms at onset. Autonomic signs are common, as are changes in mood and affect.

C. ANTERIOR FRONTOPOLAR REGION. Anterior frontopolar seizure patterns include forced thinking or initial loss of contact and adversive movements of head and eyes, with possible evolution, including contraversive movements and axial clonic jerks, and falls and autonomic signs.

D. ORBITOFRONTAL. The orbitofrontal seizure pattern is one of complex partial seizures with initial motor and gestural automatisms, olfactory hallucinations and illusions, and autonomic signs. Automatisms may include unformed or formed speech (including expletives) and walking around the room.

E. DORSOLATERAL. Dorsolateral seizure patterns may be tonic or, less commonly, clonic with versive eye and head movements and speech arrest.

F.   OPERCULAR. Opercular seizure characteristics include mastication, salivation, swallowing, laryngeal symptoms, speech arrest, epigastric aura, fear, and autonomic phenomena. Simple partial seizures, particularly partial clonic facial seizures, are common and may be ipsilateral. If secondary sensory changes occur, numbness may be a symptom, particularly in the hands. Gustatory hallucinations are particularly common in this area.

G. MOTOR CORTEX. Motor cortex epilepsies are mainly characterized by simple partial seizures, and their localization depends on the side and topography of the area involved. In cases of the lower preRolandic area there may be speech arrest, vocalization or dysphasia, tonic-clonic movements of the face on the contralateral side, or swallowing. Generalization of the seizure frequently occurs. In the Rolandic area, partial motor seizures with march or "Jacksonian" seizures occur, particularly beginning in the contralateral upper extremities. In the case of seizures involving the paracentral lobule, tonic movements of the ipsilateral foot may occur, as well as contralateral leg movements. Postictal paralysis is frequent.

H. KOJEWNIKOW'S SYNDROME. This syndrome represents a particular form of Rolandic partial epilepsy in both adults and children and is related to a variable lesion of the motor cortex. Its principal features are: (a) motor partial seizures, always well localized; (b) often late appearance of myoclonus in the same site where somatomotor seizures occur; (c) an EEG with normal background activity and a focal paroxysmal abnormality (spikes and slow waves); (d) occurrence at any age in childhood and adulthood; (e) frequently demonstrable etiology (tumor, vascular); and (f) no progressive evolution of the syndrome (clinical, electroencephalographic or psychologic, except in relation to the evolution of the causal lesion).

I. RASMUSSEN'S ENCEPHALITIS. In this condition, a previously normal child, usually about 6 to 10 years old, rapidly develops therapy-resistant focal seizures, usually motor or sensory-motor, with a slowly progressive motor deficit implicating the same cerebral hemisphere. A mild or moderate mental deficit appears later. EEG shows prominent and persistent arrhythmic delta waves, loss of "background" features, and abundant spikes. Later, seizures may implicate widely separate portions of the same hemisphere. Pathologic specimens may show gliosis, inflammation, or spongioform changes. The disease may progress to death, stabilize, or improve over time.

C. Parietal Lobe Seizures

1. General Characteristics

Parietal lobe epilepsy syndromes usually are characterized by simple partial and secondarily generalized seizures (reviewed in Chapter 2). Most seizures remain simple and exhibit sensory phenomena. Most frequently, seizures are of the anterior parietal subtype.

2. EEG Characteristics

Interictal EEGs may show: (a) normal results; (b) focal slowing; (c) focal spikes and sharp waves which are unilateral or bilateral, synchronous or asynchronous. Slow and sharp activity spreading beyond parietal leads is not uncommon.

3. Subtypes

A. ANTERIOR PARIETAL SEIZURES. Such seizures involve the posterior central gyrus and are predominantly sensory with positive or negative phenomena. Positive phenomena may include: tingling, a feeling of electricity, desire to move a body part, sensation a body part is being moved, tongue and/or facial sensations, and pain. Negative phenomena include: loss of muscle tone, numbness, a feeling that a body part is absent, or loss of awareness of a part or one-half of the body (asomatognosia).

The parts most frequently involved are those with the largest cortical representation (hand, arm, face), and seizures may spread along the posterior central gyrus producing a "Jacksonian" march of symptoms as adjacent structures are progressively effected.

B. POSTERIOR PARIETAL SEIZURES. Such seizures are frequently accompanied by prominent staring and relative immobility. Visual phenomena may occur, including formed hallucinations and metamorphopsia (visual distortions) and confusion.

C. INFERIOR PARIETAL SEIZURES. Such seizures may demonstrate severe vertigo and disorientation in space as well as abdominal sensations.

D. PARACENTRAL SEIZURES. Such seizures may demonstrate contralateral genital sensations or rotary or postural motor activity, and have a tendency to become secondarily generalized.

E. DOMINANT HEMISPHERE PARIETAL SEIZURES. Seizures arising from the dominant parietal lobe may demonstrate receptive or conductive language disturbances.

F. NONDOMINANT HEMISPHERE PARIETAL SEIZURES. Metamorphopsia and asomatognosia often indicate involvement of the nondominant parietal lobe.

D. Occipital Lobe Seizures

1. General Characteristics

Occipital lobe seizures are characterized by visual phenomena, especially elementary (nonformed) visual hallucinations (generally contralateral to the side of the seizure focus) and incomplete or complete loss of sight. Other occipital seizure manifestations include: tonic and clonic eye deviation, head deviation, blinking, a sensation of eye movement, and nystagmoid eye movements. Eye and head movements usually are contralateral to the side of the seizure focus in occipital seizures (may not be the case for seizures arising in other areas).

2. EEG Characteristics

Surface EEGs most often demonstrate extensive posterior temporal-occipital paroxysmal activity. This pattern may be difficult to distinguish from temporal lobe epilepsy of posterior temporal origin.

3. Subtypes

Seizure discharges within the occipital lobe produce a limited number of signs and symptoms. However, such discharges may spread to the temporal, frontal, supplementary motor, or parietal areas and produce seizures typical of these areas. Visual signs or symptoms at onset suggest occipital origin.

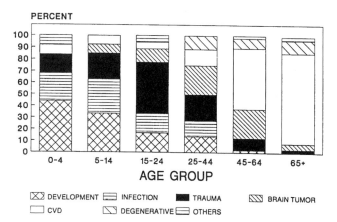

Fig. 3-1. Etiologies of symptomatic epilepsy in various age groups. From ref. (2) with permission.

E. Etiology of Partial Seizures and Localization-Related Epilepsies

1. Overall

By definition, these epilepsies are symptomatic of a cerebral lesion. The usual etiologies are developmental defects, trauma, cerebrovascular disease, tumors, and infection. The incidence of these etiologies varies with age (see Fig. 3-1).

2. Neuropathologic Examination of Temporal Lobectomy Specimens

Temporal lobectomy has been a recognized therapy for refractory epilepsy of temporal lobe origin for several decades (see Chapter 10). Neuropathologic examinations of surgical specimens provide an insight into the etiologies of such epilepsies.

Mesial temporal sclerosis is the most common finding, being present in approximately one-half of patients. Mesial temporal sclerosis refers to the pathologic entity of hippocampal sclerosis and atrophy (often visable on imaging studies) with loss of neurons in the CA1 region and end-folium (CA3/CA4), but with relative sparing of the CA2 region. Loss of dentate hilar neurons (end-folium sclerosis) is a common feature, and in some patients, may be the only apparent hippocampal lesion. The etiology of mesial temporal sclerosis is controversial. There is evidence that prolonged seizures, including prolonged febrile seizures, may cause mesial temporal sclerosis.

Congenital lesions (principally *hamartomas, heterotopias,* and *focal cortical dysplasia*) account for 15% to 20% of recognized lesions and are particularly common in children. See Kuzniecky, et al. for details (13). *Neoplasms* (principally glial) account for 10% to 15% of recognized lesions. *Trauma* accounts for only 5% to 10% of pathologic findings.

See review of Spencer (20) for more details.

F. Management of Partial Seizures and Localization-Related/Symptomatic Epilepsies

1. Seizure First Aid and Prevention of Complications

A. GENERAL. The first responsibilities of a person present with a seizing patient are to prevent physical injury, to ensure safety, and to observe accurately. Never leave the patient alone. Call for help if needed.

B. COMPLEX PARTIAL SEIZURES. Prevent falls caused by loss of tone or incoordination. Patients exhibiting automatisms (walking, standing, smoking) should be monitored. Physical restraint should only be used as a last resort because patients demonstrating automatisms may become violent if restrained.

C. TONIC-CLONIC SEIZURES. Placing a soft oral airway in the patient's mouth will prevent oral trauma and promote drainage of secretions. This should be done *only* if the airway can be placed without force (usually impossible because the mouth closes tightly early in the tonic phase). Forcing an airway between teeth will result in oral trauma. Falling patients should be caught before hitting the floor. Hands or other soft objects can be used to prevent trauma to the head or other parts, caused by clonic movements. Patients should be placed in the lateral decubitus or prone position as soon as possible to promote drainage of secretions and to prevent aspiration. Complications of tonic-clonic seizures (oral trauma, head trauma, stress fractures, aspiration pneumonia, pulmonary edema—see Chapter 2) should be looked for as soon as possible.

2. Pharmacologic Management

A. BASIC APPROACH AND PHARMACOLOGIC PRINCIPLES. See Chapter 10.

B. DRUGS OF CHOICE. The drugs of first choice in adults are carbamazepine and phenytoin, based upon comparative trials. Gabapentin, lamotrigine, and topiramate are the authors' second-choice drugs, based upon lesser risk of toxicity and drug interactions when compared with other available agents (phenobarbital, primidone, valproic acid). Drug selection in adults is discussed in more detail in Chapter 10 and a review by Mattson et al. (16). In children, comparative studies have demonstrated that carbamazepine, phenytoin, and valproic acid are equally efficacious. Phenobarbital and primidone are also efficacious, but side effects such as irritability, hyperactivity, and lethargy limit these drugs to second-line therapy.

C. DRUG ADMINISTRATION. The administration of drugs used in children and adults is presented in Tables 11-2 and 11-3. See Chapter 11 for further details on these drugs.

3. Medically Refractory Epilepsy

A. DEFINITION. Patients with localization-related/symptomatic epilepsy who continue to have seizures after trials of three or more marketed antiepileptic drugs following principles outlined in Chapter 10 are considered "medically refractory." Approximately 15% of patients with localization-related/symptomatic epilepsy (partial seizures) fall into this category. The probability that a fourth drug will completely control seizures is less than 10%. Therefore, such patients require re-evaluation of their diagnosis and management.

B. DIAGNOSTIC RE-EVALUATION. Many cases of "medically refractory" epilepsy are caused by improper diagnosis. The patient should be re-evaluated by the treating physician or a neurologic consultant to re-examine the differential diagnostic alternative diagnoses discussed in Chapter 9. Psychogenic seizures and absence seizures are the most common causes of improper diagnosis.

C. ALTERNATIVE THERAPIES.

SURGICAL MANAGEMENT. Surgical management should be considered first because the probability that a fourth drug will completely control seizures is less than 10%. The probability that a resection procedure will completely control seizures is greater that 50% in patients meeting criteria for such procedures. See Chapter 10 for full discussion.

OTHER THERAPIES. Experimental antiepileptic drugs [see Fisher and Blum (8)], behavior therapy [see Wolf (25)] and hormone therapy [see Morrell (18)] are other alternatives for patients who are not surgical candidates.

Surgery and other alternative treatments generally are available only at specialized epilepsy centers.

G. Prognosis of Partial Seizures and Localization-Related/Symptomatic Epilepsies

1. First Unprovoked Seizure

The risk of seizure recurrence by 36 months is 25% in persons with no risk factors after having a first unprovoked seizure. In persons having risk factors, the risk of seizure recurrence usually is much greater. Risk factors include: evidence of prior neurologic insult (history, neurologic examination, imaging studies), abnormal EEG, and multiple seizures or status epilepticus as initial event. Treatment of first partial seizures remains controversial because of uncertainty regarding risk of another seizure and side effects of antiepileptic medication. However, randomized clinical trials do indicate antiepileptic drugs reduce risk of seizure recurrence.

2. After Two or More Unprovoked Seizures

Persons with two or more unprovoked seizures almost always are treated. The two Veterans Adminstration Cooperative Studies (17) indicate 35–60% of adult patients with partial seizures will have complete seizure control after 1 year with carbamazepine or phenytoin monotherapy as initial and only treatment.

Satisfactory results (acceptable number or no seizures, acceptable side effects) are obtained in approximately 70% of patients with a single drug, either the initial choice or an alternative. Thirty percent of patients will have inadequate control despite trials of several drugs used alone. When a second drug is added another 10% are satisfactorily controlled. With a third drug, another 5% are satisfactorily controlled. Approximately 15% of patients are not controlled after trials of three or more drugs. Such patients are considered medically refractory.

Risk factors for poor control of partial seizures include: abnormal EEG, evidence of a structural brain lesion, number and duration of seizures prior to diagnosis and prior to control with medication, neurologic deficit from birth, and secondarily generalized tonic-clonic seizures.

3. Successful Medication Withdrawal after Remission

See Chapter 10.

4. Mortality

A. GENERAL. Available studies are not optimal but generally report increased mortality in patients with symptomatic epilepsies. This mortality is caused by, at least in part, the underlying symptomatic disease (congenital malformations, tumors, cerebrovascular disease) and its complications. Studies regarding increased rate of suicide are conflicting.

B. SUDDEN UNEXPLAINED DEATH. The risk of sudden unexplained death is approximately 4 times greater in persons with symptomatic epilepsy (but not idiopathic epilepsy) than the general population. Postulated mechanisms include cardiac arrhythmias, pulmonary edema, and suffocation. Death often occurs during sleep in adults 20 to 40 years of age with long-standing epilepsy. Other risk factors include: (1) tonic-clonic seizures; (2) low-plasma concentrations of antiepileptic drugs; and (3) cerebrovascular disease.

5. Neuropsychologic Function

Animal studies suggest repeated partial seizures may result in neuronal damage. Human studies are difficult to evaluate because of confounding effects of original structural lesion, antiepileptic drug effects, and impaired social adjustment. The effects of repeated partial seizures on neuropsychologic function remain an unanswered question.

REFERENCES

1. Acharya JN, Wyllie E, Luders H, et al. Seizure symptomatology in infants with localization-related epilepsy. *Neurology* 1997;48:189–196.
2. Annegers JF. The epidemiology of epilepsy. In: Wyllie E, ed. *The treatment of epilepsy: principles and practice*, 2nd ed. Baltimore: Williams and Wilkins, 1997.
3. Burgerman R, Sperling M, French J, et al. Comparison of mesial versus neocortical onset temporal lobe seizures: neurodiagnostic findings and surgical outcome. *Epilepsia* 1995;30:662–670.
4. Cockerall OC, Johnson AL, Sander WAS, et al. Prognosis of epilepsy: a review and further analysis of the first nine years of the British National Practice Study of Epilepsy, a prospective population-based study. *Epilepsia* 1997;38:31–46.
5. Commission on Classification and Terminology of the International League Against Epilepsy. Proposal for

revised clinical and electroencephalographic classification of epileptic seizures. *Epilepsia* 1981;22:489–501.

6. Commission on Classification and Terminology of the International League Against Epilepsy. Proposal for revised classification of epilepsies and epileptic syndromes. *Epilepsia* 1989;30:389–399.

7. Engel J, Pedley TA, eds. *Epilepsy: a comprehensive textbook.* Philadelphia: Lippincott–Raven, 1997, Chaps. 13,29,45–50,229–237.

8. Fisher R, Blum D. Clobazam, tiagabine, topiramate, and other new antiepileptic drugs. *Epilepsia* 1995;36 (Suppl 2):S105–S114.

9. French JA, Williamson PD, Thadani VM, et al. Characteristics of mesial temporal lobe epilepsy: I. results of history and physical examination. *Ann Neurol* 1993;34:774–780.

10. Gastaut H. Generalized convulsive seizures without local onset. In: Vinken PJ, Bruyn GW, eds. *Handbook at clinical neurology, Vol 15, The epilepsies.* Amsterdam: Elsevier, 1974.

11. Hauser WA. The natural history of seizures. In: Wyllie E, ed. *The treatment of epilepsy: principles and practice,*2nd ed. Baltimore: Williams and Wilkins, 1997.

12. Ho SS, Berkovic SF, Newton MR, et al. Parietal lobe epilepsy: clinical features and localization by ictal SPECT. *Neurology* 1994;44:2277–2284.

13. Kuzniecky RI, Barkovich AJ. Pathogenisis and pathology of focal malformations of cortical development and epilepsy. *J Clin Neurophysiol* 1996;13: 468–480.

14. Laskowitz DT, Sperling MR, French JA, et al. The syndrome of frontal lobe epilepsy: characteristics and surgical management. *Neurology* 1995;45:780–787.

15. Leestma JE, Annegers JF, Brodie MJ, et al. Sudden unexplained death in epilepsy: observations from a large clinical development program. *Epilepsia* 1997; 38:47–55.

16. Mattson RH. Selection of antiepileptic drugs. In: Levy RH, Mattson RH, Meldrum BS, eds. *Antiepileptic drugs,* 4th ed. New York: Raven Press, 1995.

17. Mattson RH and the V.A. Epilepsy Cooperative Studies No. 118 and 264 Group. Prognosis for total control of complex partial and secondarily generalized tonic-clonic seizures. *Neurology* 47: 68–76, 1996.

18. Morrell MJ. Hormones, reproductive health, and epilepsy. In: Wyllie E, ed. *The treatment of epilepsy:*

principles and practice, 2nd ed. Baltimore: Williams and Wilkins, 1997.

19. Salanova V, Morris HH, Van Ness P, et al. Frontal lobe seizures: electroclinical syndromes. *Epilepsia* 1995;36:16–24.

20. Spencer S. Temporal lobectomy: selection of candidates. In: Wyllie E, ed. *The treatment of epilepsy: principles and practice*, 2nd ed. Baltimore: Williams and Wilkins, 1997.

21. Sveinbjornsdottir S, Duncan JS. Parietal and occipital lobe epilepsy: a review. *Epilepsia* 1993;34:493–521.

22. Theodore WH, Porter RJ, Albert P, et al. The secondarily generalized tonic-clonic seizure: a videotape analysis. *Neurology* 1994;44:1403–1407.

23. Van Passchen W, Connelly A, King MD, et al. The spectrum of hippocampal sclerosis: a quantitative magnetic resonance imaging study. *Ann Neurol* 1997;41:45–51.

24. Wyllie E, (ed). *The treatment of epilepsy: principles and practice*, 2nd ed. Baltimore, Williams and Wilkins, 1997. (Contains series of reviews of seizure types and of the epilepsies in adults).

25. Wolf P. Behavioral therapy. In: Engel J, Pedley TA, eds. *Epilepsy: a comprehensive textbook*. Philadelphia: Lippincott–Raven, 1997.

EPILEPSIES WITH NEONATAL ONSET (BIRTH–2 MONTHS)

TABLE 4-1. *Epilepsies and epilepsy syndromes with neonatal onset (birth–2 months) and accompanying seizure types*

I. Both localization-related and generalized epilepsies
  A. Neonatal seizures syndrome (CLON, MYO, TON)
  B. Benign familial neonatal seizures syndrome (CLON)
  C. Benign neonatal convulsions syndrome (CLON)

CLON = clonic seizures; MYO = myoclonic seizures; TON = tonic seizures.

The type of seizures and epilepsy described in this chapter are both localization-related and generalized (see Chapter 1). Three syndromes may occur. These are listed in Table 4-1 which serves as an outline of this chapter.

I. BOTH LOCALIZATION-RELATED AND GENERALIZED EPILEPSIES

A. Neonatal Seizures

Neonatal seizures are one of the most common, yet ominous neurologic signs in newborns. Since seizures may be the first and only sign of a central nervous system disorder, their recognition is extremely important. Despite recent advances made in the areas of obstetrics and perinatal care, seizures continue to be a significant predictor of poor neurologic outcome.

There are a multitude of changes in neuronal and glial growth and differentiation, myelination, and neurochemical composition of the brain during the third trimester of pregnancy and postnatal months. Because of immaturities in anatomic, chemical, and bio-electric connections in and between cortical and subcortical structures, it is not surprising that neonatal seizures differ markedly from those occurring in older subjects. They differ mainly in their clinical manifestations, in their etiologies, and in their short- and long-term prognosis.

1. Definition

While there is not a rigid definition, neonatal seizures refer to seizures which occur between birth and 2 months of age.

2. Seizure Phenomena

There is a considerable difference in the behavior observed during seizures in neonates from the behaviors seen in older children and adults. Infants are unable to sustain organized generalized epileptiform discharges, and generalized tonic-clonic and absence seizures are rarely, if ever, seen. The age-dependent clinical and electroencephalogram (EEG) features in neonates are a result of the immaturity of cortical organization and myelination.

Neonatal seizures are classified as clonic, tonic, and myoclonic. *Clonic seizures* consist of rhythmic jerking of groups of muscles and occur in either a focal or multifocal pattern. In multifocal clonic seizures, movements may migrate from one part of the body to another. Although focal seizures may be seen with localized brain insults, such as neonatal strokes, they may also be seen in disorders that diffusely affect the brain such as asphyxia, subarachnoid hemorrhage, hypoglycemia, or infection. In *tonic seizures* the infant develops asymmetrical posturing of the trunk or deviation of the eyes to one side. *Myoclonic seizures* are similar to those seen in older children, consisting of rapid jerks of muscles. The myoclonic seizures can consist of bilateral jerks, although occasionally, unilateral or focal myoclonus can occur.

Sick neonates often display repetitive, stereotyped behavior that may be confused with seizures. These behaviors include repetitive sucking and other oral-buccal-lingual movements, assumption of an abnormal posture, pedaling movements of the legs or paddling movements of the arms, blinking, momentary fixation of gaze with or without eye deviation, nystagmus, or apnea. However, when these behaviors are observed during EEG recordings, epileptiform activity is usually not recorded. Likewise, when tonic posturing involves all four extremities and the trunk, there is rarely an associated EEG-epileptiform discharge. Myoclonus not associated with epileptiform discharges can also be seen in sick neonates.

3. EEG Phenomena

While the diagnosis of seizures relies primarily on clinical observation, the EEG may be extremely valuable in confirming the presence of epileptic seizures. In addition, the EEG is very useful in the detection of electrographic seizures in paralyzed infants or in assessing response to antiepileptic medications.

A. INTERICTAL ABNORMALITIES. As with older children and adults, interictal spikes are seen more frequently in infants with seizures than those without seizures. However, differentiating "normal" spikes and sharp waves from those with pathologic significance may be difficult. Strict criteria for differentiating normal sharp waves and spikes from those that are pathologic have yet to be established. For example, frontal sharp waves that shift from hemisphere to hemisphere (often termed "frontal sharp transients") and multifocal spikes and sharp waves that only occur during the burst phase of discontinuous sleep, are considered normal by many electroencephalographers. In addition, normal infants, both term and preterm, may have infrequent, sporadic spikes and sharp waves.

Criteria used to classify spikes and sharp waves as abnormal include: spikes and sharp waves that are focal and persist through all sleep states; Rolandic-positive sharp waves; and focal or multifocal spikes during the low amplitude phase of discontinuous sleep. Pathologic spikes often occur in bursts. As with older children, spikes and sharp waves can be seen in neonates who never have detected seizures.

Positive spikes occurring over the Rolandic area are often associated with underlying white matter disease, such as periventricular leukomalacia or intraventricular hemorrhages. Positive Rolandic spikes typically are not associated with seizures.

B. ICTAL DISCHARGES. Epileptiform . activity that is rhythmic and has a distinct beginning and ending is considered an ictal event. In addition, most ictal discharges have some degree of evolution in frequency or morphology of the waveforms. While there is not yet a consensus on the minimum length of time required for the discharge to be considered ictal, we define an EEG ictus as 10 sec of rhythmic epileptiform activity.

Ictal epileptiform activity can be divided into four basic types: focal spike or sharp wave discharges, focal low frequency discharges, focal rhythmic discharges, and multifocal discharges. While the type of ictal discharge has not been shown to be specific for etiology, the use of this classification system is useful for description purposes. *Focal spike or sharp wave discharges* consist of rhythmic spikes or sharp waves that originate focally. The frequency of the discharge usually exceeds 2 Hz, and spread of the focal discharge to other regions occasionally occurs. The spread of ictal discharges in the immature brain is usually much slower than in older children and adults. *Focal low frequency discharges* consist of focal spikes or sharp waves that occur at a low frequency (approximately 1 Hz). Differentiating this ictal discharge from periodic lateralized epileptiform discharges (PLEDs) is based primarily on evolution and duration. PLEDs demonstrate no evolution, typically last over 10 min, and are considered nonepileptic activity. Focal low frequency ictal discharges usually demonstrate an evolution during the discharge in regards to frequency, amplitude, or waveform morphology (Fig. 4-1). *Focal rhythmic patterns* consist of rhythmic, monomorphic waves varying from 0.5 to 15 Hz. The ictal patterns often vary in frequency during the course of the discharge. In some patients the ictal discharges "migrate" from one area of the cortex to another (Fig. 4-2A–C). The discharge may have a resemblance to "normal" activity and has been referred to as focal pseudo-beta-alpha-theta-delta discharges. However, unlike the normal background activity seen on the neonatal EEG, ictal beta-alpha-theta-delta discharges are paroxysmal, rhythmic and usually monomorphic in character. *Multifocal patterns* consist of EEG discharges originating independently, or, rarely, simultaneously from two or more foci.

Focal epileptiform activity does not necessarily imply focal pathology. Infants may have focal epileptiform discharges in the face of systemic disorders such as hypoglycemia or hypoxic-ischemic injuries. Cerebral infarctions are frequently associated with focal seizures and lateralized epileptiform discharges in term infants.

EEG seizures often occur without any clear clinical accompaniment. In general, EEG seizures without clinical accompaniment have a poorer prognosis than electrical seizures with clinical changes.

4. Differential Diagnosis

A challenge to the clinician in evaluating the neonate with seizures is differentiating seizures from other stereotyped repetitive behavior in the neonate. Many infants with central nervous system disorders will have episodes of chewing, repetitive sucking, and other oral-buccal-lingual movements, assumption of an abnormal posture, pedaling movements of the legs or paddling movements of the arms, blinking, momentary fixation of gaze with or without eye deviation, or nystagmus that is not seizure activity. The EEG is enormously helpful in helping to distinguish seizure from nonseizure activity.

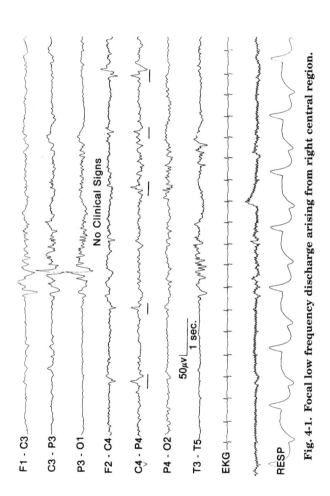

Fig. 4-1. Focal low frequency discharge arising from right central region.

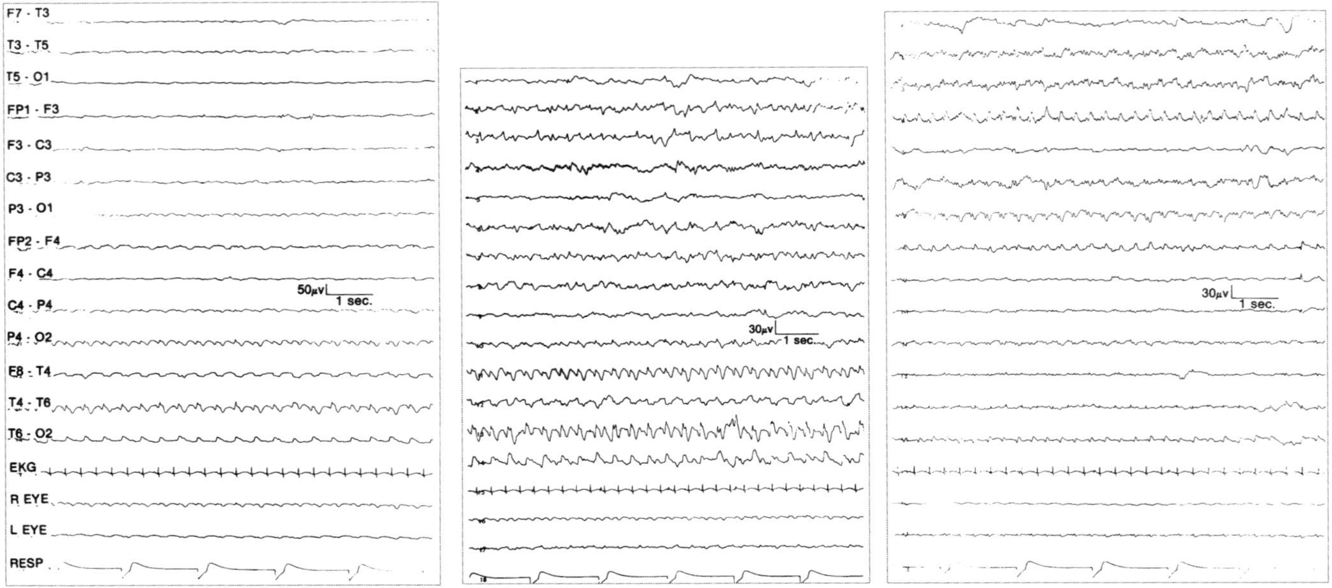

Fig. 4.2. A–C: Focal rhythmic pattern on EEG of infant with neonatal seizures. Note how the discharges "migrate" from the right temporal region area to the left. No clinical signs were observed with the seizures.

Benign neonatal sleep myoclonus is a condition in which infants during the first few months of life develop myoclonic jerks only during sleep. The EEG is very useful in differentiating benign neonatal sleep myoclonus from seizure-related myoclonus. In the former, the myoclonic jerks during sleep are not associated with any epileptiform discharges.

5. Etiology

Many seizures are the result of insults occurring before, during, or after birth. The seizures may be the response to a transient metabolic or systemic disorder. Etiologic factors are usually readily identifiable at this age, and less than one-third of neonatal seizures are cryptogenic or idiopathic in origin. Outcome correlates best with the etiologic factors rather than the frequency, severity, and duration of the seizures, in contrast with what occurs in older subjects.

Neonatal seizures require a prompt evaluation for etiology. While neonatal seizures are rarely life-threatening, the underlying condition can lead to serious neurologic impairment if not treated. For example, the neonate with meningitis benefits greater from treatment of the meningitis than treating the seizures.

Table 4-2 lists the common etiologies of neonatal seizures.

6. Management

The first step in the evaluation should be a careful history and physical examination. A family history of neonatal seizures is suggestive of benign familial neonatal seizures (see following), while a history of maternal drug ingestion may implicate drug withdrawal as a cause of seizures. Maternal infections or a difficult delivery may be helpful in determining etiology. Chorioretinitis or a skin rash may suggest a congenital infection such as toxoplasmosis, while needle marks in the scalp would raise the possibility of inadvertent injection of a local anesthetic such as lidocaine during delivery.

Following the history and physical examination, the appropriate diagnostic studies should be performed, and treatment for the seizures begun. While the history and clinical examination will dictate those studies most appropriate, in most cases, venous blood should be obtained for a complete blood count, glucose, electrolytes, ammonia, liver-function tests, bilirubin, and culture. If metabolic disease is suspected, arterial blood gases,

Table 4-2. *Etiologic agents associated with neonatal seizures*

Etiology	Comments
Asphyxia	Hypoxic-ischemic encephalopathy is most common cause of neonatal seizures.
Hypocalcemia	Hypocalcemia has two major peaks of incidence in the newborn. The first occurs during the first 3 days of life and is associated with prenatal morbidity or perinatal insults. Late-onset hypocalcemia (5 to 14 days) occurs primarily in term infants consuming a nonhuman milk preparation with a suboptimal ratio of phosphorus to magnesium. Hypomagnesemia may accompany or occur independently of hypocalcemia.
Hypoglycemia	Most authors cite glucose levels less than 20 mg/dl in preterm infants and 30 mg/dl in term babies as indicating hypoglycemia. Like hypocalcemia, hypoglycemia is often associated with other neonatal disorders.
Hyponatremia/ hypernatremia	Hyponatremia, like hypocalcemia, usually occurs in association with other disorders. Hypernatremia is usually iatrogenic, most frequently secondary to improper mixing of formula.
Intracranial hemorrhages	Although many subarachnoid hemorrhages are mild and inconsequential except for causing transient seizures, some result in a stormy course with hydrocephalus and brain parenchymal damage. Intraventricular hemorrhage is the most common type of intracranial hemorrhage and accounts for a large percentage of morbidity and mortality primarily, but not exclusively, in preterm infants.
Congenital infection	Intrauterine or postnatal central nervous system infections may lead to seizures. Intrauterine causes include rubella, toxoplasmosis, cytomegalovirus, herpes simplex, human immunodeficiency virus (HIV) and coxsackievirus B. Intrauterine infections are usually associated with other systemic signs: microcephaly, jaundice, rash, hepatomegaly, and chorioretinitis.
Postnatal infection	Common postnatal infections include *E. coli* and group B beta-hemolytic *Streptococcus*. Any infant without a clear etiology of seizures requires prompt lumbar puncture. Sepsis without meningitis may also lead to seizures.

serum amino acids, and urine organic acids should be obtained. A spinal-fluid examination is almost always indicated if the etiology of the seizures is not known.

All infants with suspected seizures should have an EEG, especially the paralyzed infant who cannot demonstrate abnormal movements. The EEG may confirm that stereotyped behavior is associated with electrical discharges. Conversely, if the behavior in question is not associated with EEG changes, the need for antiepileptic drugs may be eliminated.

Table 4-2. Continued

Etiology	Comments
Congenital malformation	Virtually all disorders of neuronal migration and organization, i.e., polymicrogyria, neuronal heterotopias, lissencephaly, holoprosencephaly, and hydranencephaly, may lead to severe neonatal seizures.
Metabolic disorders	Although the differential diagnosis of neonatal seizures includes inherited metabolic disorders these are rare and usually produce other significant symptoms such as peculiar odors, protein intolerance, acidosis, alkalosis, lethargy, or stupor. In most cases of metabolic disease, pregnancy, labor, and delivery are normal. While food intolerance may be the earliest indication of a systemic abnormality, seizures are commonly the first specific clue to central nervous system involvement. If untreated, metabolic disorders commonly lead to lethargy, coma, and death. In surviving infants, weight loss, poor growth, and failure to thrive are common.
Drug withdrawal	A significant cause of neonatal seizures in urban hospitals is withdrawal from narcotic-analgesics, sedative-hypnotics, and alcohol. Infants born to heroin- or methadone-addicted mothers have an increased risk of seizures, although the most common neurologic findings are jitteriness and irritability. Infants of methadone-addicted mothers may have late withdrawal symptoms, with seizures occurring as long as 4 weeks after birth. Maternal use of cocaine has been associated with neonatal seizures.
Inadvertent injections	Although rare, seizures may be a prominent feature in infants poisoned with local anesthetics. Inadvertent fetal anesthetic injection usually occurs in deliveries at the time of local anesthesia administered for episiotomy. The infant presents at birth with bradycardia, apnea, and hypotonia. Seizures usually occur within the first 6 hr and are generally tonic in type. The infants may have mydriasis and loss of lateral eye movements and pupillary light reflexes.

7. Treatment

The decision to treat or not to treat is usually based on a number of factors, including duration and frequency of seizures, associated autonomic dysfunction such as hypertension or apnea, etiology, and EEG abnormalities. Unfortunately, it is not yet known whether the treatment of neonatal seizures alters prognosis. However, since outcome is related to etiology, it is essential that the cause of the seizure be identified and treated, if possible.

If seizures are brief and not associated with autonomic dysfunction the clinician may decide not to treat or to treat with a short-acting benzodiazepine. Conversely, infants with frequent seizures, especially if they interfere with ventilation, require prompt and vigorous treatment.

Despite significant advances in the treatment of epilepsy in older children and adults, treatment of neonatal seizures remains unsatisfactory. Phenobarbital and phenytoin are the primary drugs used in neonates, despite the lack of convincing efficacy studies. Loading with 20 mg/kg of phenobarbital results in a serum level of approximately 20 µg/ml. It is recommended that the phenobarbital be given in two 10 mg/kg boluses, with each bolus administered over 5 min (2 to 3 mg/kg/min). If seizures persist, giving additional phenobarbital may be helpful. Phenytoin is typically used if phenobarbital is not effective and, like phenobarbital, is administered in two boluses of 10 mg/kg. While hypotension and cardiac arrhythmias rarely occur in neonates with phenytoin administration, it is recommended that each bolus of phenytoin be given at a rate no faster than 2 mg/kg/min. This loading dosage of 20 mg/kg results in blood levels of 15 to 20 µg/ml.

Infants requiring oral maintenance of antiepileptic drugs are given phenobarbital 5 mg/kg/day. Because of increasing clearance of phenobarbital with age, trough-serum levels of the drug should be checked monthly, or more frequently if seizures continue. The combination of slow and incomplete absorption, in combination with rapid clearance of the drug make it extremely difficult to administer phenytoin orally.

Other drugs, including diazepam, lorazepam, primidone, carbamazepine, lidocaine, and paraldehyde have been tried in the treatment of neonatal seizures. However, there is little information regarding the efficacy of additional drugs after metabolic abnormalities are corrected, ventilation and perfusion are satisfactory, and loading with phenobarbital and phenytoin is complete.

8. Prognosis

By far the most significant factor in determining prognosis is the etiology of the seizures. For example, infants with seizures secondary to congenital brain malformations, hypoxia-ischemia, or postnatal meningitis do far worse than infants with seizures secondary to small subarachnoid hemorrhages or transient hypocalcemia.

The EEG is a powerful prognostic tool in neonates with seizures. For prognostic purposes, the background EEG patterns are more significant than the patterns of EEG epileptiform discharges. Infants with frequent or prolonged seizures generally have a poorer outcome than those infants with infrequent seizures. However, exceptions do occur. Infants with benign familial neonatal seizures and benign neonatal convulsions often have very frequent seizures, but have an excellent prognosis. Finally, infants with normal neurologic examinations at the time of discharge from the newborn unit do better than those with abnormal examinations.

B. Benign Familial Neonatal Seizures

Unlike in older children, few epileptic syndromes have been described in neonates. This is because most neonatal seizures are not epilepsy but are reactions to acute insults. However, two syndromes have been described: benign familial neonatal seizures and benign neonatal convulsions.

The diagnosis of benign familial neonatal seizures in a neonate with seizures is based on five criteria: (a) normal neurologic examination; (b) negative evaluation for another etiology of the seizures; (c) normal developmental and intellectual outcome; (d) positive family history of newborn or infantile seizures with benign outcome; and (e) onset of seizures during the neonatal or early infantile period. Although most infants have seizures during the first week of life, a small percentage of patients have a later onset. This disorder has been linked to chromosome 20 and represents one of the few legitimate epileptic syndromes of the neonate.

The seizures are usually frequent for a few days then stop. The infant is usually alert and vigorous between the seizures. Clonic seizures, focal or multifocal, are the most frequent seizure type, although generalized seizures have been reported. The seizures are generally brief, lasting for approximately 1 to 2 min, but may occur as often as 20 to 30 times a day.

The interictal EEG is of little assistance in making the diagnosis of benign familial neonatal seizures since it may or may not be abnormal. No specific diagnostic features have been reported. When abnormal, the findings are frequently transient. Ictal records are characterized by an initial flattening on the EEG followed by bilateral discharges of spikes and sharp waves. This condition may represent a generalized seizure disorder.

C. Benign Neonatal Convulsions

Benign neonatal convulsions, also called benign neonatal idiopathic seizures, are characterized by seizures occurring in term, otherwise healthy infants. The seizures are usually partial clonic in type, and may be confined to one body part or migrate from one region to another. Apnea may occur with the clonic activity or be the sole manifestation of the seizure. The seizures often escalate into a crescendo of activity. Initially, the patient is normal between the seizures. The seizures then increase in frequency until the child goes into status epilepticus. The flurry of seizures usually lasts less than 24 hr, although less frequent seizures may continue for a few days.

A search for etiology is not revealing. While the seizures may be very frequent, they usually resolve after a few days. Since the seizures often begin on the fifth day of life, some authors have described these seizures as "fifth day fits."

Like benign familial neonatal seizures, EEG findings in benign, idiopathic neonatal seizures have been variable. An EEG pattern felt to be associated with this syndrome has been described. The "theta pointu alternant" pattern consists of dominant theta activity, which is discontinuous, unreactive, often asynchronous, and has intermixed sharp waves. However, the theta pointu alternant pattern is not specific for benign seizures and can be seen following a variety of neonatal encephalopathies.

Both benign familial neonatal seizures and benign neonatal convulsions are diagnoses of exclusion. Even with a positive family history of benign neonatal seizures, other more ominous disorders should be ruled out.

REFERENCES

1. Engel J, Pedley TA, eds. *Epilepsy: a comprehensive textbook*. Philadelphia: Lippincott–Raven, 1997, Chaps. 12,55–57,117,213–215.
2. Hirsch E, Velez A, Sellal F, et al. Electroclinical signs of benign neonatal familial convulsions. *Ann Neurol* 1993;34:835–841.
3. Holmes GL. Neonatal seizures. *Sem Pediatr Neurol* 1994;1:72–82.

4. Holmes GL, Lombroso CT. Prognostic value of background patterns in the neonatal EEG. *J Clin Neurophysiol* 1993;10:323–352.
5. Lombroso CT, Holmes GL. Value of EEG in neonatal seizures. *J Epilepsy* 1993;6:39–70.
6. Miles DK, Holmes GL. Benign neonatal seizures. *J Clin Neurophysiol* 1990;7:369–379.
7. Mizrahi EM. Consensus and controversy in the clinical management of neonatal seizures. *Clin Perinatol* 1989;16:485–500.
8. Mizrahi EM, Kellaway P. Characterization and classification of neonatal seizures. *Neurology* 1987;37:1837–1844.
9. Painter MJ, Bergman I, Crumrine P. Neonatal seizures. *Pediatr Clin North Am* 1986;33:91–109.
10. Painter MJ, Gaus LM. Neonatal seizures: diagnosis and treatment. *J Child Neurol* 1991;6:101–108.
11. Painter J, Pippenger C, Wasterlain C, et al. Phenobarbital and phenytoin in neonatal seizures: metabolism and tissue distribution. *Neurology* 1981;31:1107–1112.
12. Petit RE, Fenichel GM. Benign familial neonatal seizures. *Arch Neurol* 1991;37:47–48.
13. Rowe JC, Holmes GL, Hafford J, Baboval D, et al. Prognostic value of the electroencephalogram in term and preterm infants following neonatal seizures. *Electroencephalogr Clin Neurophysiol* 1985;60:183–196.
14. Rust RS, Volpe JJ. Neonatal seizures. In: Dodson WE, Pellock JM, editors. *Pediatric epilepsy: diagnosis and therapy*. New York: Demos Publications, 1993:107–128.
15. Wyllie E, ed. *The treatment of epilepsy: principles and practice*, 2nd ed. Baltimore: Williams and Wilkins, 1997, Chaps 6,9,40,86.

EPILEPSIES WITH ONSET DURING INFANCY (2-12 MONTHS)

TABLE 5-1. *Epilepsies and epilepsy syndromes with onset during infancy (2–12 months) and accompanying seizure types.*

I. Localization-related/symptomatic epilepsies
   A. Temporal lobe epilepsy syndromes (SPS, CPS, TCS)
   B. Frontal lobe epilepsy syndromes (SPS, CPS, TCS)
   C. Parietal lobe epilepsy syndromes (SPS, CPS, TCS)
   D. Occipital lobe epilepsy syndromes (SPS, CPS, TCS)
II. Generalized/symptomatic epilepsies
   A. West syndrome (infantile spasms) (spasm)
   B. Tonic seizures (TON)
   C. Atonic seizures (ATO)
   D. Lennox-Gastaut syndrome (TON, TCS, MYO, ABS, ATO)
III. Generalized/either idiopathic or symptomatic
   A. Benign myoclonic epilepsy of infancy (MYO)
   B. Severe myoclonic epilepsy of infancy (MYO, SPS, TCS, ABS)
   C. Myoclonic-astatic epilepsy syndrome (MYO, ATO)
IV. Situation related epilepsies
   A. Febrile convulsions (TCS, TON)

ABS = absence seizures; ATO = atonic seizures; CPC = complex partial (psychomotor, temporal lobe) seizures; MYO = myoclonic seizures; SPS = simple partial (focal) seizures; TCS = tonic-clonic (grand mal) seizures; TON = tonic seizures

The epilepsies and epilepsy syndromes with onset during infancy (2–12 months) and accompanying seizure types are listed in Table 5-1. This table also serves as an outline for this chapter.

I. LOCALIZATION-RELATED/SYMPTOMATIC EPILEPSIES

Localization-related/symptomatic epilepsies can occur at any age. Three seizure types occur with these epilepsies: simple partial (focal), complex partial (psychomotor, temporal lobe) and tonic-clonic (grand mal). The clinical and EEG features of these three seizure types are reviewed in Chapter 2. Differential diagnostic entities to consider in children and adults when diagnosing these seizures types, are listed in Chapter 2 and reviewed in Chapter 9.

Depending on locus of onset, four groups of localization-related/symptomatic epilepsy syndromes have been recognized (Table 5-1). Clinical and EEG features, management and prognosis of these four syndromes are reviewed in Chapter 3.

II. GENERALIZED/SYMPTOMATIC EPILEPSIES

The four disorders discussed in this section (West syndrome, tonic seizures, atonic seizures, and Lennox-Gastaut syndrome) are true age-dependent epileptic conditions. West syndrome and Lennox-Gastaut syndrome always begin during early childhood, while the vast majority of patients with tonic and atonic seizures have seizure onset during the first year of life.

These conditions are classified as generalized seizures, since the clinical and EEG features typically suggest widespread involvement of the cortex. However, in many of the patients the seizures have a partial onset with rapid secondary generalization.

A. West Syndrome (Infantile Spasms)

Clinical and EEG features of seizures in children vary as a function of age. A good example of these age-related phenomena is infantile spasms, a unique seizure disorder confined to early childhood. Infantile spasms are an age-specific disorder occurring only in children during the first 2 years of life. The peak age of onset is between 4 and 6 months of age, and approximately 90% of infantile spasms begin before 12 months of age.

1. Definition

The characteristic features of this syndrome are myoclonic seizures, hypsarrhythmic electroencephalograms, and mental retardation. This triad is sometimes referred to as *West syndrome*. As will be seen, however, not all cases conform strictly to this definition. The disorder is also referred to in the literature as massive spasms, salaam seizures, flexion spasms, jackknife seizures, massive myoclonic jerks, and infantile myoclonic seizures.

2. Seizure Phenomena

Infantile spasms may vary considerably in their clinical manifestations. Some seizures are characterized by brief head nods while other seizures consist of violent flexion of the trunk, arms, and legs. The diagnosis may often be delayed since the parents and even the family physician may not recognize spasms as seizures. What is usually not variable is that in each child the spasms are stereotyped. In addition, spasms characteristically occur in flurries.

While resembling a myoclonic or tonic seizure, the spasm is a distinct type of seizure. A myoclonic jerk is a rapid shocklike contraction of limited duration, while the tonic seizure is a prolonged muscle contraction of growing intensity. The true spasm consists of a characteristic muscular contraction that lasts from 1 to 2 seconds, and reaches a peak more slowly than a myoclonic jerk, but more rapidly than a tonic seizure.

The seizures in infantile spasms are of three types: flexor, extensor, and mixed flexor-extensor. *Flexor spasms* consist of brief contractions of flexor musculature of the neck, trunk, arms, and legs. Spasms of the muscles of the upper limbs result either in adduction of the arms in a self-hugging motion, or in abduction of the arms to either side of the head with the arms flexed at the elbow. *Extensor spasms* consist predominantly of extensor muscle contractions, producing abrupt extension of the neck and trunk with extensor abduction or adduction of the arms, legs, or both. *Mixed flexor-extensor spasms* include flexion of the neck, trunk, and arms and extension of the legs, or flexion of the legs and extension of the arms with varying degrees of flexion of the neck and trunk. Asymmetric spasms occasionally occur and resemble a "fencing" posture. Infantile spasms are frequently associated with eye deviation or nystagmus.

Asymmetric spasms can be seen when the muscular contractions do not occur simultaneously on the two sides of the body. This type of spasm is usually observed in symptomatic infants with severe brain lesions or agenesis of the corpus callosum, or both. Focal signs, such as eye or head deviation, may accompany symmetric and asymmetric spasms. Asymmetric spasms generally are isolated, but can also follow a partial seizure or precede a partial seizure, or sometimes appear simultaneously with a partial or generalized seizure.

Infantile spasms frequently occur in clusters, and the intensity and frequency of the spasms in each cluster may increase to a peak before progressively decreasing. The seizures are very brief, and single seizures may be missed by the casual observer. The number of seizures per cluster varies considerably, with some clusters having as many as 150 seizures. Number of clusters per day also varies, with some patients having as many as 60 clusters per day. Clusters can occur at night, although they rarely occur during sleep. Crying or irritability during or after a flurry of spasms is commonly observed.

3. EEG Phenomena

Infantile spasms are associated with markedly abnormal EEGs. The most commonly seen *interictal pattern* is *hypsarrhythmia*, which consists of very high voltage, random, slow waves and multifocal spikes and sharp waves (Fig. 5-1). The chaotic appearance of the EEG abnormality gives the impression of total disorganization of cortical voltage and rhythms. During sleep, there are bursts of polyspike and slow waves. Somewhat surprising, in view of the marked background abnormalities, is the persistence of sleep spindles in some patients. During rapid eye movement (REM) sleep there may be a marked diminution or complete disappearance of the hypsarrhythmic pattern. Infantile spasms are associated with a decrease of the total sleep time, as well as a decrease in REM sleep. Variations in hypsarrhythmia have been described, including patterns with: interhemispheric synchrony, a consistent focus of abnormal discharge, episodes of attenuation, and high-voltage slow activity with few sharp waves or spikes. The variant patterns of hypsarrhythamia are frequent and do not correlate with prognosis.

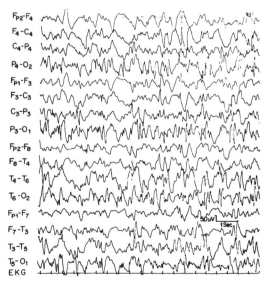

Fig. 5-1. Example of hypsarrhythmic EEG from infant with infantile spasms.

Although a hypsarrhythmic or modified hypsarrhythmic pattern is the most common type of interictal abnormality seen in infantile spasms, this EEG pattern may not be present in some patients with infantile spasms. Some patients with infantile spasms do not have hypsarrhythmia early in the course of the disorder, but go on to develop the pattern. Although hypsarrhythmia is primarily associated with infantile spasms, it occurs in other disorders as well.

Like the interictal pattern, the *ictal EEG* changes during infantile spasms are variable. The most characteristic ictal EEG pattern of the spasms consists of a positive wave over the vertex-central region; low amplitude fast (14 to 16 Hz) activity or a diffuse flattening, called decremental activity, may also be seen.

The presence of focal features is one of the variations of the basic hypsarrhythmic patterns and may be associated with partial seizures. Partial seizures may precede, accompany, or follow the cluster of spasms. This observation suggests that cortical "pacemakers" may be important in the development of infantile spasms.

EEGs are not static in this disorder and may evolve over time. Some patients with spasms may not have hypsarrhythmia at the onset of their disorder. Other patients may have slow EEG recordings with rare epileptiform activity that then develop into hypsarrhythmic patterns. Follow-up EEG recordings may be necessary to demonstrate hypsarrhythmia.

4. Basic Mechanisms

The clinical and ictal EEG features of infantile spasms are suggestive of a generalized seizure disorder. Yet, as will be seen, some children with infantile spasms will respond to surgical removal of a cortical lesion. For that reason the brainstem, which has widespread projections throughout the central nervous system, has been implicated as playing an important role in the genesis of infantile spasms. An underlying disruption of neuronal function within specific nuclei of the pontine reticular formation could result in interference with descending pathways that exert control over spinal reflexes and result in infantile spasms. In addition, the hypsarrhythmic EEG pattern could be the result of abnormal input to the thalamic and cortical neurons through ascending projections.

5. Differential Diagnosis

Because infantile spasms differ significantly from the clinical features of other seizures in young children, it is not surprising that parents and primary caretakers may miss the diagnosis. Unfortunately, the pediatrician or family physician rarely has the opportunity to actually see the spasms and has to depend on the description by the parents. With increasing use of home videotaping and greater awareness of the problem, delay to diagnosis is being reduced. Occasionally, the clinical course will be atypical, and the spasms will not occur in clusters, or involve only slight movements or episodes of akinesia. In these patients, the EEG will be helpful since it is invariably abnormal.

There are a few other conditions that may be confused with infantile spasms. *Early myoclonic epileptic encephalopathy (EMEE)* and *early infantile epileptic encephalopathy (EIEE)* are syndromes that have a clinical similarity to infantile spasms. EMEE is characterized clinically by the occurrence of sporadic and erratic fragmentary myoclonus, usually in association with other seizure types. The EEG demonstrates burst-suppression. A variety of etiologic agents has been associated with the disorder including metabolic diseases, cerebral dysgenesis, and hypoxic-ischemic insults. The prognosis in the disorder is severe, with most infants dying within a year or having severe neurologic sequelae.

EIEE, also termed *"Ohtahara's syndrome,"* is a disorder with onset in early infancy, with severe, frequent tonic seizures, and a burst-suppression pattern on the EEG. The infants have severe developmental deficits and may evolve into West syndrome. As with EMEE, infants with the disorder have had a host of associated etiologies, including cerebral dysgenesis.

Benign nonepileptic infantile spasms is a syndrome which begins in infancy with the flexion spasms. However, the syndrome differs from West syndrome by the absence of mental retardation or regression, and the presence of normal EEGs both during wakefulness and sleep.

Benign neonatal sleep myoclonus, which was discussed under neonatal seizures, may be confused with infantile spasms. The EEG is very helpful in distinguishing the two conditions.

6. Etiology

On the basis of past history, physical examination, and laboratory studies, cases of infantile spasms have been conventionally classified into those in which there is no apparent preceding neurologic disorder or identified etiologic factor (*idiopathic*), and those in which a pre-existing presumptively responsible pathologic event or disorder is demonstrated (*symptomatic* cases). Some authors use another category, *cryptogenic*, to refer to children with developmental delay or an abnormal neurologic examination before the onset of spasms, but in whom an etiology cannot be determined.

As can be seen in Table 5-2, infantile spasms has been associated with a wide variety of etiologies. Virtually any disorder that can cause brain damage can be associated with infantile spasms. *Tuberous sclerosis* is associated with a high incidence of infantile spasms. In three large series of patients with tuberous sclerosis, 42% of the patients had a history of infantile spasms. Conversely, in reports of cases of infantile spasms, the frequency of patients with tuberous sclerosis has varied from 4% to 25%. Tuberous sclerosis is difficult to diagnose during the first year of life because the characteristic skin lesion, adenoma sebaceum, never occurs before the age of 3 years. However, infants may have hypopigmented areas on the skin which may only be detectable using a Wood's lamp. If the diagnosis is suspected, further evidence for the disorder may come from a computerized axial tomography (CAT) scan which may demonstrate intracranial calcifications, abdominal ultrasound which may detect polycystic kidneys, and an echocardiogram which may demonstrate cardiac tumors. The magnetic resonance imaging (MRI) may show cortical tubers, although calcium is not seen well using this technique.

Aicardi's syndrome should be considered in girls with infantile spasms. In addition to infantile spasms, girls have absence or partial absence of the corpus callosum, dorsal vertebral anomalies, and chorioretinal lacunar defects. The ocular lesions are frequently associated with colobomas of the optic nerve and microphthalmia. The syndrome appears to be X-linked, occurring primarily in girls.

A controversy exists as to whether the pertussis immunization can lead to infantile spasms. The vaccine is given at the time of peak incidence of infantile spasms, and, therefore, a temporal coincidence would be expected in a large number of cases. In addition, it is often difficult to determine the exact time of onset of the spasms. However, when closely documented cases are reviewed, the link between the pertussis vaccine and infantile spasms is

Table 5-2. Etiologic factors associated with infantile spasms

Prenatal	Perinatal	Postnatal
Congenital cerebral anomolies:	Hypoxic-ischemic encephalopathies	Metabolic disturbances:
Hydrocephalus	Meningitis	Nonketotic hyperglycinemia
Microcephaly	Encephalitis	Maple syrup urine disease
Hydranencephaly	Trauma	Phenylketonuria
Schizencephaly	Intracranial hemorrhages	Phenylketonuria
Polymicrogyria		Mitochondrial
Sturge-Weber		Meningitis
Incontinentia pigmenti		Encephalitis
Tuberous sclerosis		Degenerative disease
Down syndrome		
Aicardi's syndrome		
Hypoxic-ischemic encephalopathies		
Congenital infections		
Trauma		

quite weak. It remains possible that in a small number of children, especially in cases where a striking neurologic reaction occurs within 24 hr after the immunization, that a causal relation exists. It is also possible that in some cases, the vaccine acts in conjunction with other unidentified factors to precipitate the clinical onset of symptoms in children already predisposed to the disease. A recently developed acellular pertussis vaccine appears to significantly reduce the risk of adverse events associated with the vaccine.

The finding that some infants have infantile spasms while others with similar brain disturbances do not, suggests that genetic susceptibility may be important.

7. Management

The infant that presents with infantile spasms requires a thorough evaluation which includes a developmental assessment, neurologic examination, and laboratory studies to try to determine an etiology. In addition, the neurologic and developmental examinations at the time of diagnosis are important indicators of prognosis.

The skin should be closely inspected for hypopigmented lesions which can occur in tuberous sclerosis. These lesions often cannot be seen unless the infant is examined with a Wood's lamp in a darkened room.

Laboratory studies ordered will be determined largely by the history and physical examination. Every child with the possible diagnosis should have an EEG and neuroimaging. A normal EEG would raise questions about the diagnosis and suggest that the child has benign myoclonus of early infancy.

A CAT or MRI scan is recommended in every patient with infantile spasms since it may provide valuable information regarding the etiology. For example, cranial calcifications may indicate tuberous sclerosis or a congenital infection. In addition, brain anomalies such as agenesis of the corpus callosum, porencephaly, and hydranencephaly will be apparent on the CAT or MRI scan. Abnormal neuroimaging occurs in 70% to 80% of patients with infantile spasms. The most common abnormality seen in large series has been diffuse cerebral atrophy.

Because pyridoxine dependency has been associated with infantile spasms in children in whom an etiology cannot be definitely established, an infusion of 100 to 200 mg pyridoxine intravenously during EEG monitoring may be useful. Infants with pyridoxine dependency should have an improvement in the seizures and EEG within minutes.

Infants who do not have an adequate explanation for the seizures should undergo a metabolic evaluation. This will include urine and serum amino acid screening, serum ammonia, organic acid, lactate, pyruvate, and liver-function tests. A spinal-fluid examination should include glucose (which should be compared to a serum glucose level), protein, and cell count. Cerebrospinal fluid (CSF), amino acids, pyruvate, and lactate should be obtained in children when metabolic disease is suspected. Since most children will be placed on corticotropin (ACTH), electrolytes, calcium, phosphorus, glucose, and urine analysis should be obtained.

8. Treatment

A. ACTH AND CORTICOSTEROIDS. Corticotropin and corticosteroids are the primary drugs used in the treatment of infantile spasms, although studies using vigabatrin appear quite promising. Vigabatrin had not yet received FDA approval for use in the United States at the time this book went to press.

The effects of ACTH and other therapies on long-term outcome remain controversial. For example, several authors have found no developmental differences between patients who did or did not receive treatment. For the large number of infants who exhibit pre-existing brain damage, it is unlikely that any form of therapy would greatly influence the long-range outcome in terms of mental and motor development. The important question is whether the type of treatment for infantile spasms in children who were normal before the onset of the spasms, or who have a cryptogenic cause of the spasms, alters outcome. The majority of evidence suggests that treatment with ACTH results in a lower incidence of seizures and better psychomotor development than treatment with oral steroids, such as prednisone, or other antiepileptic drugs.

The dosage and length of time a child should be treated with ACTH or corticosteroids has not been established. In view of the lack of consensus regarding dosage and treatment duration, the following approach is necessarily empiric. The recommended starting dose of ACTH is 40 IU/day given intramuscularly. A nonsynthetic form of ACTH gel should be used. If the seizures do not completely resolve by 2 weeks, the dose should be increased by 10 IU increments every week until the seizures cease or a daily dosage of 80 IU is reached. The ACTH is given for a minimum of 1 month following the cessation of seizures. At that time a taper can begin, decreasing by 10 units a week. It the seizures persist despite a maximum dose of ACTH, a trial of valproic acid or nitrazepam is recommended. If relapse occurs during the taper or after discontinuation of ACTH, the ACTH should be restarted at the dose that originally stopped the spasms. Following control of the seizures, the ACTH should be continued for a minimum of 1 month before tapering is attempted again. The response to ACTH is sometimes very dramatic with cessation of seizures and marked improvement of the EEG within a few days.

While ACTH and corticosteroids can be very effective in stopping spasms, it can result in many side effects, some of which can be very serious. Steroid therapy is invariably associated with cushingoid obesity. In addition, growth retardation, acne, and irritability may ensue. In the short-term use of ACTH, these side effects are of no major concern. More serious side effects include infection, arterial hypertension, intracerebral hemorrhages, osteoporosis, gastrointestinal bleeding, hypokalemic alkalosis, and other electrolyte disturbances.

Children treated with ACTH or adrenal corticosteroids should be closely monitored. Twice-weekly blood pressure measurements and checks on stool guaiac as well as periodic checks of electrolyte levels should be performed. If the child develops hypertension or hypokalemic alkalosis, a reduction in dosage is recommended. However, patients who have a relapse once the dosage is decreased may be restarted on the effective dose and managed with antihypertensives and/or salt restriction. If this is not effective, it is prudent to change to synthetic glucocorticoids (methylprednisone) which have a less sodium-retaining effect. Fever should be investigated promptly.

B. VIGABATRIN. The most recent drug used to treat infantile spasms is the antiepileptic drug vigabatrin, a structural analogue of gamma-aminobutyric acid (GABA) which is a selective, enzyme-activated irreversible inhibitor of GABA-aminotransferase. An excellent response to vigabatrin among children with infantile spasms has been reported in a number of studies. Patients with both symptomatic and cryptogenic infantile spasms respond to vigabatrin. While some children relapse while on the drug, the majority of children who show an initial response to the drug continue to do well on it.

C. SURGERY. Infants with intractable infantile spasms who have evidence of focal lesions may benefit from surgery. However, it should be remembered that there are case reports of infants with focal lesions associated with infantile spasms and hypsarrhythmia who responded to medication or resolved spontaneously. Therefore, surgery should only be contemplated if antiepileptic drugs, including ACTH, are not effective. The early success of focal resections in cases of infantile spasms is a promising, new approach. However, further studies evaluating the long-term outcome of infants undergoing surgery is necessary.

9. Prognosis

Infantile spasms are one of the most devastating seizure disorders to affect infants. The poor prognosis has been confirmed in virtually all follow-up studies. A significant number of infants will demonstrate psychomotor retardation and continue to have seizures. In addition, a large number of patients have neurologic abnormalities on examination. Because a substantial majority of patients have brain injury prior to the onset of the spasms, it is not surprising that the prognosis is so poor. In all likelihood these children would have had similar neurologic outcomes, regardless of the infantile spasms.

Prognosis is directly related to etiology. Authors who have coded their cases as symptomatic and idiopathic have found that idiopathic cases have a significantly better prognosis than symptomatic cases. Cryptogenic cases have a significantly better prognoses than symptomatic cases. Patients who are classified as doubtful usually have outcomes similar to the symptomatic case.

Neurologic status prior to the onset of infantile spasms is an important prognostic factor. Children with normal neurologic examinations and development have a much better prognosis than infants with developmental delay and abnormal neurologic examinations. A poor prognostic sign reported by some authors is early onset (before 6 months). However, age of onset appears related to etiology, since the onset of the spasms is at a younger age in children with symptomatic etiologies than those with cryptogenic etiologies. The occurrence of other types of seizures, in addition to the spasms and focal interictal EEG abnormalities, have been associated with a poor prognosis. In addition, reappearance of hypsarrhythmia between consecutive spasms of a cluster has been considered a favorable feature. Finally, there is some evidence that early cessation of the spasms is of prognostic significance. Therefore, early diagnosis and treatment are important.

In some children the seizures evolve into other seizure types, such as the Lennox-Gastaut syndrome. Often, the tonic seizures in this syndrome are virtually identical to the tonic seizures seen with infantile spasms. The similarities of clinical and EEG features in the two syndromes strengthen the hypothesis that the two syndromes represent age-related manifestations of similar epileptogenic processes.

B. and C. Tonic and Atonic Seizures

1. Definitions

Tonic seizures are brief seizures consisting of the sudden onset of increased tone in the extensor muscles. If standing, the patient typically falls to the ground. Their duration is longer than myoclonic seizures. Electromyographic activity is dramatically increased in tonic seizures. Conversely, atonic seizures consist of the sudden loss of muscle tone. The loss of muscle tone may be confined to a group of muscles, such as the neck, resulting in a head drop or involve all trunk muscles, leading to a fall to the ground.

While occasionally tonic and atonic seizures can be the only types of seizure experienced by the child, the majority of children with these seizure types have the *Lennox-Gastaut syndrome,* which will be discussed briefly below and in detail in Chapter 6.

2. Seizure Phenomena

Tonic seizures frequently begin with a tonic contraction of the neck muscles, leading to fixation of the head in an erect position, widely opened eyes, and jaw-clenching or mouth-opening. Contraction of the respiratory and abdominal muscles often follows, and may lead to a high-pitched cry and brief periods of apnea. The tonic contractions may extend to the proximal musculature of the upper limbs, elevating the shoulders and abducting the arms. Asymmetric tonic seizures vary from a slight rotation of the head to a tonic contraction of all the musculature of one side of the body. Occasionally, tonic seizures terminate with a clonic phase. Eyelid retraction, staring, mydriasis, and apnea are commonly associated with the motor activity and may be the most prominent features. The seizures may cause falls and injury.

Tonic seizures are typically activated by sleep and may occur repetitively throughout the night. They are much more frequent during nonREM sleep than during wakefulness, and usually do not occur during REM sleep. During tonic seizures the patient is unconscious, although arousal from light sleep may occur. Since they are often very brief, they often go undetected. Tonic seizures are usually brief, lasting from a few seconds to a minute, with an average duration of about 10 seconds. In seizures lasting longer than a few seconds impairment of consciousness is usually apparent. Postictal impairment with confusion, tiredness, and headache is common. The degree of postictal impairment is usually related to the duration of the seizure.

Atonic seizures begin suddenly and without warning and cause the patient, if standing, to fall quickly to the floor. Since there may be total lack of tone, the child has no means to protect himself/herself and injuries often occur. The attack may be fragmentary and lead to dropping of the head with slackening of the jaw or dropping of a limb. In atonic seizures, there should be a loss of electromyographic activity. Consciousness is impaired during the fall, although the patient may regain alertness immediately upon hitting the floor.

While tonic and atonic seizures can occur at all ages and are, therefore, not as age-dependent as infantile spasms, they typically begin during childhood. While atonic seizures are common in Lennox-Gastaut syndrome, they are usually less frequent than tonic and myoclonic seizures.

3. EEG Phenomena

The interictal EEG of patients with tonic seizures is usually quite abnormal, consisting of slowing of the background, with multifocal spikes, sharp waves, and bursts of irregular spike-and-wave activity. The EEG ictal manifestations of *tonic seizures* usually consist of bilateral synchronous spikes of 10 to 25 Hz of medium to high voltage, with a frontal accentuation. Simple flattening or desynchronization may also occur. Occasionally, multiple spike-and-wave or diffuse slow activity may occur during a tonic seizure.

Atonic seizures are usually associated with rhythmic spike-and-wave complexes varying from slow, 1 to 2 Hz, to more rapid, irregular spike- or multiple spike-and-wave activity. In myoclonic-astatic seizures, the EEG pattern consists of bilaterally synchronous, regular, or irregular 2 to 3 Hz spike-and-wave, while the background activity exhibits an excess of monomorphic theta activity.

4. Basic Mechanisms

While tonic and atonic seizures are classified as generalized seizures, in some patients it is possible to detect a focal onset to the ictus which then rapidly generalizes to involve diffuse cortical structures. *Tonic seizures* often begin in the frontal lobe, thus accounting for the intense motor activity seen during these seizures. Because of the sudden loss of muscle tone, it has been surmised that *atonic seizures* involve brainstem structures.

5. Differential Diagnosis

Tonic seizures are usually not difficult to diagnose. Sometimes children with very severe encephalopathies have episodes of *opisthotonic posturing* that may resemble tonic seizures. Recording an episode usually helps distinguish the two events; tonic seizures would be associated with spike-wave discharges or a discharge of rapid spikes, while no epileptiform discharges should be seen during opisthotonic posturing.

Paroxysmal choreoathetosis is a rare, usually familial, disorder characterized by episodic attacks of severe dystonia, choreoathetosis, or both. Two types have been described: paroxysmal dystonic choreoathetosis of Mount and Reback and paroxysmal kinesigenic choreoathetosis. In paroxysmal dystonic choreoathetosis, the patient has a sudden onset of severe, often painful, dystonia that may affect the arms, legs, or trunk and speech. Consciousness is not impaired during the attacks, which last from minutes to hours, and are often precipitated by alcohol, caffeine, excitement, stress, or fatigue. The disorder is inherited through an autosomal-dominant pattern. Paroxysmal kinesigenic choreoathetosis is characterized by the sudden assumption of dystonic posturing or choreoathetosis. The kinesigenic attacks are usually shorter in duration than the dystonic form, and are frequently induced by sudden movements or a startle. These attacks can occur hundreds of times daily.

Atonic seizures and pallid infantile syncope, which is discussed in Chapter 9, may, on occasion, be confused. Spasmus nutans is a disorder occurring in toddlers which is characterized by head tilt, head nodding, and nystagmus, which is often asymmetric. The head nodding may be confused with atonic seizures. Spasmus nutans is usually a self-limiting condition, disappearing after a period of 4 months to several years.

6. Etiology

As with infantile spasms, virtually any disorder that can lead to brain damage may result in tonic and atonic seizures. Common etiologies include hypoxic-ischemic encephalopathy, head injuries, encephalitis, strokes, congenital brain anomalies, and metabolic disturbances.

7. Management

As with infantile spasms, laboratory studies ordered will be determined largely by the history and physical examination. Every child with tonic or atonic seizures should have an EEG and neuroimaging. A normal EEG would be very unusual in patients with atonic and tonic seizures, and should suggest another diagnosis. Magnetic resonance imaging scans are useful in screening for congenital brain anomalies, congenital infections, and metabolic disturbances. Patients without an adequate explanation for the seizures should also have metabolic screening. This will include urine and serum amino acid screening, serum ammonia, organic acid, lactate, pyruvate, and liver-function tests. A spinal-fluid examination should include glucose (which should be compared to a serum glucose level), protein, and cell count. Cerebrospinal fluid amino acids, pyruvate, and lactate should be obtained in children when metabolic disease is suspected.

8. Treatment

Treatment of tonic and atonic seizures present the clinician with a difficult task. Complete seizure control is rarely achieved. Because of the intractable nature of the seizures and their mixed types, there is a tendency to place the child on numerous antiepileptic drugs. This polypharmaceutical approach rarely results in good seizure control and usually causes toxic reactions — fatigue, nausea, and ataxia — from the cumulative effect of the drugs. Valproic acid, felbamate, lamotrigine, and the benzodiazepines are probably the most effective drugs used in this syndrome. The ketogenic diet should also be considered if antiepileptic drugs are not effective.

9. Prognosis

The vast majority of children with atonic and tonic seizures will have the Lennox-Gastaut syndrome. As will be seen, in general this syndrome is associated with a poor prognosis.

D. Lennox-Gastaut Syndrome

The Lennox-Gastaut syndrome is characterized by a mixed seizure disorder of which tonic seizures are a major component as well as a slow spike-and-wave EEG pattern. The syndrome always begins in childhood and is often accompanied by mental retardation. The syndrome usually has onset between infancy and age 7. It is reviewed in detail in Chapter 6.

III. GENERALIZED/EITHER IDIOPATHIC OR SYMPTOMATIC

A. Benign Myoclonic Epilepsy of Infancy

Benign myoclonic epilepsy in infancy is characterized by the occurrence of brief myoclonic seizures occurring in otherwise normal infants and toddlers between the age of 4 months to 3 years. The myoclonic seizures are always brief, and usually involve the arms and head, but not the legs. The frequency and intensity of the seizures is variable. Other seizure types do not develop.

The interictal EEG in the condition is usually normal. Myoclonic jerks are associated with generalized spike-and-wave or polyspike-and-wave activity. The frequency of the discharges is greater than 3 Hz and usually last 1 to 3 sec. Some bursts of spike-and-wave activity may rarely occur during the awake state without any accompanying clinical changes. Photosensitivity occurs in some of the patients. Some patients will have generalized spike-and-wave discharges only during sleep. Sleep organization appears to be normal.

B. Severe Myoclonic Epilepsy of Infancy

Severe myoclonic epilepsy in infancy is a disorder that typically begins during the first year of life as a febrile seizure that is either generalized or unilateral. The febrile seizures tend to be long and recurrent. Between 1 and 4 years of age, the child develops myoclonic seizures. Partial seizures often occur as well. Psychomotor development is typically delayed from the second year of life and ataxia, corticospinal tract dysfunction, and non-epileptic myoclonus may occur. The epilepsy is very resistant to all forms of treatment and the children are mentally retarded.

At the time of the first febrile seizure, the EEG is usually normal and without any paroxysmal abnormalities. Between ages 1 and 2 years the myoclonic seizures begin. The myoclonus can be massive, involving whole muscles, particularly the axial one, or be barely discernible. The jerks can be isolated or occur in flurries. During EEG monitoring, generalized spike-and-wave or polyspike-and-wave activity is seen during the seizures. When absence seizures occur they are also associated with generalized spike-and-wave, usually at a frequency of 3 Hz. The generalized discharges increase during drowsiness. Focal and multifocal spikes and sharp waves are also seen.

C. Myoclonic-Astatic Epilepsy Syndrome

Atonic attacks may be associated with myoclonic jerks either before, during, or after the atonic seizure. This combination has been described as *myoclonic-astatic seizures*, also known as *Doose syndrome*. In this syndrome, astatic (defined as the inability to stand) seizures occur suddenly, without warning, and the child collapses onto the floor as if his or her legs had been pulled from under. No apparent loss of consciousness accompanies these seizures. At times, the astatic seizures are so short that only a brief nodding of the head and slight flexion of the knees is seen. The myoclonic seizures in this disorder are characterized by symmetric jerking of the arms and shoulders, with simultaneous nodding of the head. Some myoclonic jerks are violent, with the arms flung upward; some are so mild that they are easier to feel than see. A combination of myoclonic and astatic seizures is frequently observed. In these children, the loss of postural tone is immediately preceded by myoclonic jerks; hence, the term "myoclonic-astatic seizures."

The onset of the disorder takes place between the first and fifth year of age and occurs in boys more frequently than girls. With few exceptions, the mental and motor development of the children is normal before the onset of the disorder. However, in some children, the prognosis is unfavorable and dementia may occur. Absence status is reported to play a role in the pathogenesis of the dementia.

IV. SITUATION RELATED EPILEPSIES
A. Febrile Convulsions

Febrile convulsions usually occur between ages 6 months and 5 years. Febrile convulsions are reviewed in Chapter 8.

REFERENCES

1. Alvarez LA, Shinnar S, Moshé SL. Infantile spasms due to unilateral cerebral infarcts. *Pediatrics* 1987; 79:1024–1026.
2. Chiron C, Dulac O, Luna D, et al. Vigabatrin in infantile spasms. *Lancet* 1990;335:363–364.
3. Chiron C, Dulac O, Beaumont D, Palacios L, Pajot N, Mumford J. Therapeutic trial of vigabatrin in refractory infantile spasms. *J Child Neurol* 1991;6(Suppl. 2):2S52–2S59.
4. Chugani HT, Shewmon A, Shields WD, Sankar R, Comair Y, Vinters HV, et al. Surgery for intractable infantile spasms: neuroimaging perspectives. *Epilepsia* 1993;34:764–771.
5. Dalla Bernardina B, Fontana E, Sgrò V, Colamaria V, Elia M. Myoclonic epilepsy ('myoclonic status') in nonprogressive encephalopathies. In: Roger J, Bureau M, Dravet C, Dreifuss FE, Perret A, Wolf P, eds. *Epileptic syndromes in infancy, childhood and adolescence*. 2nd ed. London: John Libbey, 1992:89–96.
6. Donat JF, Wright FS. Seizures in series: similarities between seizures of the West and Lennox-Gastaut syndromes. *Epilepsia* 1991;32:504–509.
7. Dravet C, Bureau M, Genton P. Benign myoclonic epilepsy of infancy: electroclinical symptomatology and differential diagnosis from the other types of generalized epilepsy on infancy. In: Degen R, Dreifuss FE, eds. *Benign localized and generalized epilepsies of early childhood*. Amsterdam: Elsevier Science, 1992:131–135.
8. Dravet C, Bureau M, Guerrini R, Giraud N, Roger J. Severe myoclonic epilepsy in infants. In: Roger J, Bureau M, Dravet C, Dreifuss FE, Perret A, Wolf P, eds. *Epileptic syndromes in infancy, childhood and adolescence*. 2nd ed. London: John Libbey, 1992:75–88.
9. Doose H. Myoclonic-astatic epilepsy. In: Degen R, Dreifuss FE, eds. *Benign localized and generalized epilepsies of early childhood*. Amsterdam: Elsevier Science Publishers, B.V. 1992:163–168.
10. Doose H, Baier WK. Epilepsy with primarily generalized myoclonic-astatic seizures: a genetically determined disease. *Eur J Pediatr* 1987;146:550–554.

11. Egli M, Mothersill I, O'Kane M, O'Kane F. The axial spasm—the predominant type of drop seizure in patients with secondary generalized epilepsy. *Epilepsia* 1985;26:401–415.

12. Engel J, Pedley TA, eds. *Epilepsy: a comprehensive textbook.* Philadelphia: Lippincott–Raven, 1997, Chaps. 12,53–56,216–219.

13. Holmes GL. Myoclonic, tonic, and atonic seizures in children. *J Epilepsy* 1988;1:173–195.

14. Holmes GL, Vigerano F. Infantile spasms. In: Engel J, Pedley TA, eds. *Epilepsy: a comprehensive textbook.* Philadelphia: Lippincott–Raven, 1997.

15. Jeavons PM, Livet MO. West syndrome: infantile spasms. In: Roger J, Bureau M, Dravet C, Dreifuss FE, Perret A, Wolf P, eds. *Epileptic syndromes in infancy, childhood and adolescence.* 2nd ed. London: John Libbey, 1992:1–65.

16. Ikeno T, Shigematsu H, Miyakoshi M, Ohba A, Yagi K, Seino M. An analytic study of epileptic falls. *Epilepsia* 1985;26:612–621.

17. Kellaway P, Hrachovy RA, Frost JD, Jr., Zion T. Precise characterization and quantification of infantile spasms. *Ann Neurol* 1979;6:214–218.

18. Koo B, Hwang PA, Logan WJ. Infantile spasms: Outcome and prognostic factors of cryptogenic and symptomatic group. *Neurology* 1993;43:2322–2327.

19. Kramer V, Sue WC, Mikati M: Hypsarrhythmia: Frequency of variant patterns and correlation with etiology and outcome. *Neurology* 1997;48:197–203.

20. Lombroso CT. A prospective study of infantile spasms: clinical and therapeutic considerations. *Epilepsia* 1983;24:135–158.

21. Snead OC, III., Benton JW, Myers GL. ACTH and prednisone in childhood seizure disorders. *Neurology* 1983;33:966–970.

22. Wyllie E, ed. *The treatment of epilepsy: principles and practice*, 2nd ed. Baltimore: Williams and Wilkins, 1997, Chaps. 35–37,41.

EPILEPSIES WITH CHILDHOOD ONSET (1–12 YEARS)

TABLE 6-1. *Epilepsies and epilepsy syndromes with onset during childhood (1–12 years) and accompanying seizure types*

I. Localization-related/symptomatic epilepsies
  A. Temporal lobe epilepsy syndromes (SPS, CPS, TCS)
  B. Frontal lobe epilepsy syndromes (SPS, CPS, TCS)
  C. Parietal lobe epilepsy syndromes (SPS, CPS, TCS)
  D. Occipital lobe epilepsy syndromes (SPS, CPS, TCS)
II. Localization-related/idiopathic epilepsies
  A. Benign childhood epilepsy with centrotemporal spikes (SPS, CPS, TCS)
  B. Childhood epilepsy with occipital paroxysms (SPS, CPS, TCS)
III. Generalized/idiopathic epilepsies
  A. Childhood absence epilepsy (ABS, TCS)
  B. Juvenile absence epilepsy (ABS, TCS)
  C. Juvenile myoclonic epilepsy (MYO, TCS, ABS)
  D. Epilepsy with tonic-clonic seizures on awakening (TCS)
  E. Epilepsy with random tonic-clonic seizures (TCS)
IV. Generalized/symptomatic epilepsies
  A. Lennox-Gastaut syndrome (TON, TCS, MYO, ABS, ATO)
V. Generalized/either idiopathic or symptomatic
  A. Generalized tonic-clonic seizures (TCS)
  B. Progressive myoclonic seizures (MYO, TCS, CLO)
  C. Myoclonic-akinetic epilepsy syndrome (MYO, ATO)
VI. Situation-related epilepsies
  A. Febrile convulsions (TCS, TON)
  B. Seizures with special modes of precipitation (SPS, CPS, TCS, MYO, ABS)
VII. Special syndromes
  A. Landau-Kleffner syndromes (SPS, CPS, TCS, MYO)

ABS = absence seizures; ATO = atonic seizures; CLO = clonic seizures; CPC = complex partial seizures (psychomotor, temporal lobe); MYO = myoclonic seizures; SPS = simple partial (focal) seizures; TCS = tonic-clonic (grand mal) seizures; TON = tonic seizures

The epilepsies and epilepsy syndromes with onset during childhood (1–12 years) and accompanying seizure types are listed in Table 6-1. This table also serves as an outline of this chapter.

I. LOCALIZATION-RELATED/SYMTOMATIC EPILEPSIES

Localization-related/symptomatic epilepsies can occur at any age. Three seizure types occur with these epilepsies: simple partial (focal), complex partial (psychomotor, temporal lobe) and tonic-clonic (grand mal). The clinical and electroencephalogram (EEG) features of these three seizure types are reviewed in Chapter 2; management and prognosis are reviewed in Chapter 3. Differential diagnostic entities to consider in children and adults when diagnosing these seizure types are listed in Chapter 3 and reviewed in Chapter 9.

Depending on locus of onset, four groups of localization-related/symptomatic epilepsy syndromes have been recognized (Table 6-1). Clinical and EEG features, management and prognosis of these four syndromes are reviewed in Chapter 3.

II. LOCALIZATION-RELATED/IDIOPATHIC EPILEPSIES

There are two major syndromes in which partial seizures may be a major component: benign Rolandic epilepsy and benign occipital epilepsy.

A. Benign Rolandic Epilepsy

1. Definitions and Etiology

Benign Rolandic epilepsy (BRE) is an important, distinct epileptic syndrome occurring in childhood that is characterized by nocturnal tonic-clonic seizures of probably focal onset and diurnal simple partial seizures arising from the lower Rolandic area of the cortex. The EEG pattern is characteristic, consisting of midtemporal-central spikes. It is important for the clinician to be aware of this syndrome since evaluation and prognosis differ considerably from other focal seizure disorders.

Benign Rolandic epilepsy is limited to the pediatric-age group. Seizures begin between the ages of 2 and 12 years, although more typically the child is between 5 and 10 years of age. Seizures of BRE remit spontaneously and do not occur after 16 years of age. The developmental and neurologic examination is usually normal.

The disorder is usually familial. It is inherited by a single, autosomal-dominant gene, with a low, age-dependent penetrance. Fifty percent of close relatives (siblings, children, and parents of the probands) demonstrate the EEG abnormality between the ages of 5 and 15 years. Before 5 and after 15 years of age there is a low penetrance, with few patients demonstrating the abnormality. Only 12% of patients who inherit the EEG abnormality have clinical seizures.

2. Seizure Phenomena

The syndrome is termed "Rolandic epilepsy" because of the characteristic feature of partial seizures involving the region around the lower portion of the central gyrus of Rolando. While a nocturnal tonic-clonic seizure is the most dramatic and common mode of initial presentation, diurnal simple partial seizures may also lead to a neurologic evaluation.

The characteristic features of daytime seizures include: (a) somatosensory stimulation of the oral-buccal cavity; (b) speech arrest; (c) preservation of consciousness; (d) excessive pooling of saliva; and (e) tonic or tonic-clonic activity of the face. Less often, the somatosensory sensation will spread to the face or arm. On rare occasions, a typical Jacksonian march of tonic or tonic-clonic activity will occur.

While the somatosensory aura is quite common, this history is frequently not elicited, especially in young patients. Motor phenomena during the daytime attacks are usually restricted to one side of the body and include tonic, clonic, or tonic-clonic events. These attacks most frequently involve the face, although the arm and leg may be involved. While seizures rarely generalize during wakefulness, the sensory or motor phenomenon may change sides during the course of the attack. Arrest of speech may initiate the attack or occur during its course. Consciousness is rarely impaired during the daytime attacks. Following the seizure the child may feel numbness, pins and needles, or "electricity" in his tongue, gums and cheek on one side. Postictal confusion and amnesia are unusual following seizures in BRE. In nocturnal seizures, the initial event is typically clonic movements of the mouth with salivation and gurgling sounds from the throat. Secondary generalization of the nocturnal seizure is common. The initial focal component of the seizure may be quite brief.

The seizures may occur both during the day and night, although in most children they are most common during sleep. Both the daytime and nocturnal seizures are brief. The frequency of seizures in BRE is typically low, and it is unusual for status epilepticus to develop.

3. EEG Phenomena

The disorder is characterized by a distinctive EEG pattern. The characteristic interictal EEG abnormality is a high amplitude, usually diphasic spike with a prominent, following slow wave. The spikes or sharp waves appear singly or in groups at the midtemporal (T3,T4) and central (Rolandic) region (C3,C4) (Fig. 6-1). The spikes may be confined to one hemisphere or occur bilaterally. Rolandic spikes usually occur on a normal background.

Occasional records have generalized spike-wave discharges, usually during sleep. Most children with BRE who have spike-wave discharges during sleep do not have typical absence seizures.

Sleep usually increases the number of spikes. Since approximately 30% of children with BRE have spikes only during sleep, it is important that sleep be obtained in children with the suspected syndrome. Sleep states are usually normal in BRE.

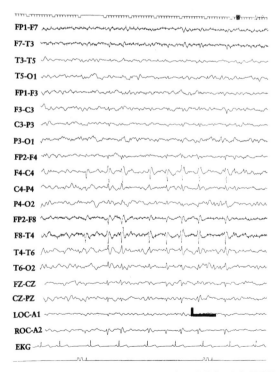

Fig. 6-1. Example of Rolandic spikes in child with BRE. Note that the spikes are present in both the right central (C4) and temporal (T4) regions.

4. Management

If the patient has a clinical history and EEG characteristics of this disorder and a normal neurologic examination, further workup is not necessary. If the neurologic examination is abnormal, or EEG demonstrates abnormalities other than the typical epileptiform discharge, further evaluation with a magnetic resonance imaging (MRI) scan is recommended.

Because of the benign nature of BRE many physicians may choose not to treat the first or second seizure. If treatment is initiated, the seizures are usually controlled with a single antiepileptic drug. Drugs used for partial seizures, i.e., phenobarbital, phenytoin, carbamazepine, and valproic acid are usually effective.

The EEG is not a good predictor of recurrence risk. Most patients can be tapered off medications after 1 to 2 years of seizure control, regardless of whether the EEG normalizes.

5. Prognosis

The prognosis of BRE is excellent, with the majority of children going into remission by the teenage years.

B. Benign Occipital Epilepsy

1. Definition

Benign occipital epilepsy (BOE) is a benign form of partial epilepsy in childhood, characterized by seizures beginning with visual ictal symptoms and interictal-occipital rhythmic EEG spikes appearing only after eye closure. The clinical and EEG features of the syndrome are stereotyped enough to warrant its inclusion as a syndrome. The peak age of onset is between 5 and 7 years of age. In some cases the disorder runs in families.

2. Seizure Phenomena

The visual symptoms consist of amaurosis, elementary visual hallucinations (i.e., phosphenes), complex visual hallucinations, or visual illusion, including micropsia or metamorphopsia. The visual symptoms occur in less than one-half of the patients with the syndrome. A variety of motor activity is seen in this disorder. Hemiclonic seizures, adversive, complex partial, and generalized tonic-clonic seizures can occur. Headaches with associated nausea and vomiting occur commonly after the seizure.

Both the clinical manifestations and frequency of the seizures are somewhat variable, depending on when the seizure occurs. In nocturnal seizures motor symptoms predominate, whereas in diurnal seizures visual symptoms are most common. Nocturnal seizures are more common in younger children and appear to bear a good prognosis. Seizures starting after the age of 8 are more likely to be frequent and diurnal, and continue for longer periods of time.

3. EEG Phenomena

The interictal EEG is characterized by normal background activity and well-defined occipital discharges. The occipital spikes are typically high in voltage (200 to 300 μV) and diphasic, with a main negative peak followed by a relatively small positive peak and a negative slow wave. An important feature in this syndrome is the prompt disappearance with eye opening and its reappearance 1 to 20 sec after eye closure.

A few words of caution regarding occipital spikes are necessary. The syndrome of BOE requires more than the EEG finding of occipital spikes. Like centrotemporal spikes, not all children with reactive occipital-spikes pattern develop seizures. Occipital spikes can also be seen in other disorders. Children with myoclonic, absence, and photosensitive epilepsies may have similar EEG findings, but would not be classified as having BOE.

4. Management

This syndrome should be differentiated from children with occipital spikes occurring both during eye opening and eye closure. These children are usually below the age of 4 years. Only approximately one-half of children with occipital spikes studied have seizures. Unlike benign epilepsy of childhood with occipital paroxysms, the seizures typically do not include visual phenomenon or postictal headaches.

5. Prognosis

Prognosis is variable. Seizure control is achieved in 60% of patients, although seizure control may be difficult in some patients. While seizures may continue into adulthood, many children outgrow their seizures.

III. GENERALIZED/IDIOPATHIC EPILEPSIES

A. Childhood Absence Epilepsy

B. Juvenile Absence Epilepsy

1. Seizure Types

Typical absence seizures (Fig. 6-2) and generalized onset tonic-clonic seizures may occur in this syndrome. The clin-

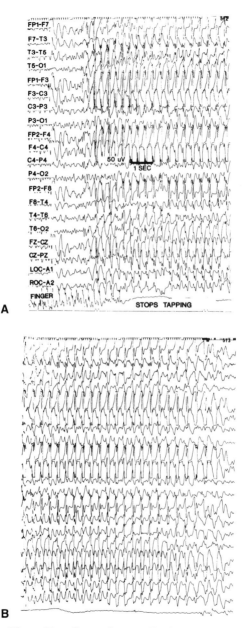

Fig. 6-2. Three Hz spike-and-wave discharge in child with typical absence seizures. Note that child quits tapping with finger shortly after onset of the spike-and-wave discharge. The child began tapping again shortly after the spike-and-wave discharge stopped.

ical and EEG features of these seizure types are reviewed in Chapter 2.

2. Other Features

In *childhood absence epilepsy (pyknolepsy)* the frequency of absence seizures is high, occurring up to several hundred times per day. *Juvenile absence epilepsy* seizure frequency is much less. In *juvenile myoclonic epilepsy*, myoclonic and generalized tonic-clonic seizures are also seen, and it is unusual for children with the syndrome to have many absence seizures. Childhood absence epilepsy usually begins between the age of 3 and puberty; juvenile absence epilepsy and juvenile myoclonic epilepsy begins during or after puberty. While generalized tonic-clonic seizures can occur in both syndromes, the incidence is higher in children with juvenile absence seizures than the childhood form.

The syndrome of *epilepsy with myoclonic absences* is characterized by absences accompanied by severe bilateral rhythmical clonic, and sometimes tonic, activity. The myoclonic movements involve mainly the muscles of the shoulders, arms, and legs. The muscles of the face are less frequently involved. Typically, there is a rhythmic and striking jerking of the shoulders, head, and arms. Tonic contractions occur in the shoulder and deltoid muscles, and result in elevation of the arms. The disorder typically begins between 5 to 10 years of age and affects boys more frequently than girls. Seizures are frequent and less responsive to medication than those of childhood absence epilepsy. Mental deterioration and evolution to Lennox-Gastaut syndrome may occur.

3. Management

Patients with suspected absence seizures do not require an extensive evaluation. Children who have typical absence seizures with consistent EEG-ictal and interictal features, and normal intelligence and neurologic examinations, require no further diagnostic tests. Patients with abnormal neurologic examinations, a history of developmental delay, or who have focal slowing or consistently focal spikes on the EEGs should have an imaging study, preferably an MRI scan.

Antiepileptic drugs are recommended for all children with adequate documentation of absence seizures. Although not life-threatening, absence seizures may lead to poor school performance and accidents. Since even brief bursts of generalized spike-and-wave discharge can affect cognitive function and responsiveness, it is prudent to try to control the seizures as quickly as possible with minimal drug toxicity.

Because absence seizures are brief and frequently subtle, their frequency can be grossly underestimated by parents. Each follow-up evaluation by the physician should include 3 to 5 minutes of hyperventilation. Activation of a seizure by hyperventilation would indicate that the patient is not under optimal control, regardless of the history supplied by the patient and parents.

Accidental injury is common with absence seizures and usually occurs after antiepileptic drug treatment is started. Injury prevention counseling is indicated. Bicycle accidents pose a special risk, and helmet use should be mandatory.

4. Treatment

The drugs of choice for typical absence seizures are ethosuximide and valproic acid. Both drugs are effective in the treatment of typical absence seizures, and a previously untreated patient on either drug has a better than 70% chance of significant reduction or total elimination of seizures. Valproic acid also has efficacy for tonic-clonic seizures (sometimes associated with absence seizures), while ethosuximide does not. A single drug should be chosen and, after appropriate laboratory studies, administered according to guidelines in Table 11-2.

Most clinicians will begin therapy with ethosuximide, primarily because of the rare, but severe, hepatotoxicity and pancreatitis associated with valproic acid. The efficacy of valproic acid is comparable to ethosuximide, and valproic acid is considered the drug of choice in the patient who has both absence and tonic-clonic seizures. Clonazepam also demonstrates efficacy in absence seizures but is usually reserved for refractory cases because of the relatively high incidence of drowsiness and behavioral side effects.

The combination of ethosuximide and valproic acid may be more effective than either drug alone, although drug interactions do occur, requiring monitoring of clinical toxicity and serum drug levels. The combination of valproic acid and clonazepam has been associated with precipitation of absence status.

The duration of therapy is variable, although a general rule is to taper patients off therapy after two seizure-free years. The EEG is very helpful in this situation, since persistence of generalized spike-and-wave discharge would indicate that there is a high likelihood of recurrence of the seizures. It is important that hyperventilation be performed during the EEG.

5. Prognosis

In general, children with absence seizures do well, with a significant proportion (65% in one study) going into remission before adulthood. Childhood absence seizures often remit by puberty, while juvenile absence seizures may persist into the late teenage years. Although it is unusual for adults to develop absence seizures, childhood-onset absences may continue into adult years. Children with juvenile myoclonic epilepsy are more likely to continue to have absence seizures into adulthood. Favorable prognostic signs for "outgrowing" absence seizures are a negative family history of epilepsy, normal EEG background activity, normal intelligence, and absence of absence status epilepticus, myoclonic seizures, or tonic-clonic seizures. Nearly 90% of children with these characteristics remit. As a general rule, onset of generalized tonic-clonic seizures prior to absence seizures, carries a poorer prognosis than the reverse order. In one study, 15% of children with absence seizures later developed juvenile myoclonic epilepsy.

Patients with atypical absences have a less favorable outlook. As will be discussed, children with atypical absences and the Lennox-Gastaut syndrome often have frequent and refractory seizures, and status epilepticus is common. The course and prognosis of epilepsy with myoclonic absences, is variable but less favorable than that of childhood absence epilepsy.

C. Juvenile Myoclonic Epilepsy

D. Epilepsy with Tonic-Clonic Seizures on Awakening

E. Epilepsy with Random Tonic-Clonic Seizures

These epilepsy syndromes may begin before the age of 12 years. However, they typically begin after the age of 12 years and are reviewed in Chapter 7.

IV. GENERALIZED/SYMPTOMATIC EPILEPSIES

A. Lennox-Gastaut Syndrome

1. Definitions

The Lennox-Gastaut syndrome (LGS) is characterized by a mixed seizure disorder (of which tonic seizures are a major component) and by a slow spike-and-wave EEG pattern. The syndrome always begins in childhood and is often accompanied by mental retardation.

The child with the LGS typically has a mixture of seizure types. The most frequently occurring are tonic, tonic-clonic, myoclonic, atypical absences, and "head drops," which represent a form of atonic, tonic, or myoclonic seizures. The syndrome is characterized by very frequent seizures, usually occurring multiple times daily.

2. Seizure Phenomenon

Tonic seizures are one of the most frequently occurring seizure types in this syndrome. They are typically activated by sleep and may occur repetitively throughout the night. They are much more frequent during non-REM sleep than during wakefulness and do not occur during REM sleep. In the LGS, tonic seizures are usually brief, lasting from a few seconds to 1 minute, with an average duration of about 10 sec. The seizures may throw the patient off balance, being responsible for many of the falls observed in children with this syndrome. Eyelid retraction, staring, mydriasis, and apnea are commonly associated and may be the most prominent features. During tonic seizures the patient is unconscious, although arousal from light sleep may occur. Since they are often very brief they usually go undetected.

3. EEG Phenomenon

The hallmark of the EEG finding in the LGS is the slow spike-and-wave discharge superimposed on an abnormal, slow background. The slow spike-and-wave or sharp-and-slow-wave complexes consist of generalized discharges occurring at a frequency of 1.5 to 2.5 Hz (Fig. 6-3). The morphology, amplitude, and repetition rate may vary both between bursts and during paroxysmal bursts of spike-and-wave activity; asymmetries of the discharge frequently occur. The area of maximum voltage, while variable, is usually frontal or temporal in location. Sleep frequently increases the frequency of the discharges, while hyperventilation and photic stimulation rarely activate these discharges.

During non-REM sleep, slow spike-and-wave discharges may be replaced by multiple-spike-and-wave discharges, whereas in REM sleep the paroxysmal activity decreases markedly. The typical EEG manifestation of tonic seizures is the occurrence of fast rhythm discharges of 10 to 20 Hz, of progressively increasing amplitude, at times followed

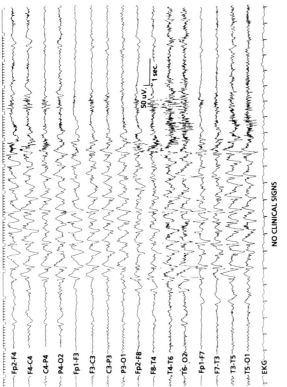

Fig. 6-3. Slow spike-and-wave discharge in a child with Lennox-Gastaut syndrome. Compare the frequency and morphology to Fig. 6-2.

by a few slow waves or spike-waves. In atonic seizures, the EEG pattern is most frequently a fast, recruiting discharge, but bursts of slow spike-wave complexes or high amplitude 10 Hz discharges are sometimes recorded. During myoclonic seizures, the EEG demonstrates bursts of irregular spike-wave activity. Atypical absence seizures are associated with slow (<2.5 Hz), often asymmetrical and irregular spike-and-wave activity.

4. Treatment

Treatment of Lennox-Gastaut syndrome presents the clinician with a formidable task. Complete seizure control is rarely achieved. Because of the intractable nature of the seizures and their mixed types, there is a tendency to place the child on numerous drugs. This polypharmaceutical approach rarely results in good seizure control and usually causes toxic reactions — fatigue, nausea, and ataxia — from the cumulative effect of the drugs.

Valproic acid, phenytoin, felbamate, lamotrigine, topiramate, and the benzodiazepines are most commonly used to treat this syndrome. Valproate has the advantage of being a broad spectrum drug with effectiveness against all of the common seizure types in the syndrome. This, coupled with the lack of sedative side effects, has prompted widespread use of the drug in this syndrome. Unfortunately, because of its association with hepatotoxicity the drug must be used cautiously in children, particularly those below the age of 2 years.

Felbamate was the first drug proven to be effective in a placebo-controlled study in the treatment of the Lennox-Gastaut syndrome. The drug was found to be effective in a number of seizure types, including atonic or drop attacks. Unfortunately, the drug was found to be associated with aplastic anemia and hepatotoxicity, and the drug is now reserved for patients who have failed other forms of therapy.

Phenytoin can be useful in the treatment of tonic and atonic seizures, although it rarely is helpful in atypical absence seizures. The benzodiazepines, such as clonazepam, also have a broad spectrum of action but are hindered by the high incidence of adverse side effects such as fatigue, irritability, and cognitive impairment. In addition, a large number of patients develop tolerance to the antiepileptic effect of the drug. While not yet rigorously studied in the Lennox-Gastaut syndrome, lamotrigine also appears to be a broad-spectrum antiepileptic drug that can be effective in a number of the seizures encountered in the Lennox-Gastaut syndrome.

While the goal of therapy should be seizure control on a single drug, most children with Lennox-Gastaut syndrome are on multiple drugs. While the efficacy of combination therapy has not been evaluated well, occasionally, polytherapy is useful in controlling seizures. The combination of lamotrigine and valproic acid has been very effective in the treatment of some children with Lennox-Gastaut syndrome.

The *ketogenic diet* is one of the oldest methods of treating childhood epilepsy. However, it remains a reasonable alternative for children with Lennox-Gastaut syndrome refractory to standard drug therapy. The diet consists of a high proportion of fats and small amounts of carbohydrate and protein. Typically, the diet consists of a fat-to-carbohydrate and protein ratio of 4:1. The basis of the therapeutic effectiveness of the ketogenic diet is felt to be the ketosis that develops when the brain is relatively deprived of glucose as an energy source and must shift to utilization of ketone bodies as the primary fuel. Modifications of this "classic" 4:1 diet have been devised in recent years, and include the medium-chain triglyceride (MCT) diet, substitution of corn oil for MCT oil, and a "modified" MCT diet consisting of a mixture of long- and medium-chain triglycerides.

Overall, the literature supports the consensus view that the ketogenic diet improves seizure control to a remarkable degree in some children. One-third to one-half of children appear to have an excellent response to the ketogenic diet in terms of a marked or complete cessation of seizures, or reduction in seizure severity. An improvement in alertness and behavior has also been reported on the diet, although this has never been subjected to scientific scrutiny. Another one-third of children have a partial or incomplete response, with some reduction in seizure frequency or severity, while the remaining one-third to one-half do not seem to benefit from the diet.

5. Prognosis

Mental retardation is present before onset of the seizures in 20% to 60% of patients. Some patients, with idiopathic or cryptogenic etiologies of their seizures, have normal intelligence quotient (IQ) scores or developmental histories before the onset of their seizures. The proportion of retarded patients increases with age because of the deterioration that frequently occurs in LGS, although rarely, a few patients escape mental retardation. Fluctuations in cognitive abilities may occur in LGS patients and are, to some degree, correlated with the intensity of EEG abnormalities. Behavioral problems are also common in LGS, ranging from hyperactivity to frank psychotic and autistic behavior. Abnormalities of the neurologic examination are common in the disorder.

Although the natural course of the disorder is for a decreasing frequency of atonic, myoclonic, and atypical absence seizures with increasing age, often there is an increase in generalized tonic-clonic seizures and an emergence of partial seizures. Sadly, only a few children undergo seizure remission.

V. GENERALIZED/EITHER IDIOPATHIC OR SYMPTOMATIC

A. Tonic-Clonic Seizures

The clinical and EEG features of tonic-clonic seizures are discussed in Chapter 2. The management of tonic-clonic seizures is discussed in Chapter 3.

B. Progressive Myoclonic Epilepsy

1. Clinical Features

Progressive myoclonic epilepsy (PME) encompasses a group of disorders in which myoclonus is a major component. In addition, the patients typically have generalized tonic-clonic or clonic seizures, mental deterioration culminating in dementia, and a neurologic syndrome which nearly always includes cerebellar dysfunction. The myoclonus involves a combination of segmental, arrhythmic, asynchronous, asymmetrical myoclonus and massive myoclonia. In addition to cerebellar symptoms, common neurologic deficits involve visual, pyramidal, extrapyramidal systems, and partial seizures, particularly those beginning in the occipital region.

Progressive myoclonic epilsepsy is usually progressive with relentless deterioration of neurologic functions and with increasing severity of the myoclonus and seizures. Almost all patients are severely ataxic, demented, wheelchair bound or bedridden. The exceptions are Unverricht-Lundborg disease and sialidosis, both of which may occur with minimal or absence of dementia. Conditions in which PME is seen include Unverricht-Lundborg disease, sialidosis, Gaucher's disease (glucocerebroside β-glucosidase deficiency), mitochondrial encephalomyopathy with ragged-red fibers (MERRF), Lafora's disease, and neuronal ceroid lipofuscinosis. For a review of these disorders the reader is referred to review articles by Berkovic and colleagues (1,2).

2. EEG Features

Even though the etiologies are different, many of the progressive myoclonic epilepsies share similar EEG findings. Typically, the alpha activity slows and is eventually replaced by theta and delta range frequencies. Epileptiform activity consists of bilateral synchronous spikes, polyspikes, spike-and-wave, or polyspike-and-wave complexes. When focal spikes are present they are most commonly seen in the occipital region. During the awake state the myoclonus may or may not be associated with spikes or spike-and-wave. During sleep, spike-and-wave discharges may decrease. The major exceptions to this rule are the sialidoses and neuronal ceroid lipofuscinosis.

While visual evoked potentials (VEPs) and brainstem auditory evoked potentials (BAEPs) are usually normal in the PMEs, somatosensory evoked potential (SSEPs) may be abnormal, demonstrating giant responses.

3. Management

Although myoclonic seizures can be seen in some benign syndromes, myoclonic seizures may be associated with a number of malignant conditions. Because of this, children with myoclonic seizures should be closely evaluated.

Once the diagnosis is established children should have an MRI seeking congenital anomalies, infections, and metabolic disturbances. Unless there is a clear etiology for the seizures the children should have metabolic screening which should include urine and serum amino acids, ammonia, lactate, pyruvate, organic acids, and liver-function tests. Spinal fluid examination should include glucose (which should be compared to a serum glucose level), protein, and cell count. Cerebrospinal fluid amino acids, pyruvate, and lactate should be obtained in children when metabolic disease is suspected. If there is a question of a mitochondrial encephalopathy, DNA testing for specific deletions and a muscle biopsy evaluating structure of the mitochondria should be performed.

4. Treatment

Myoclonic seizures may be very difficult to control. Valproic acid and the benzodiazepines are probably the most effective antiepileptic drugs used in this syndrome. The ketogenic diet should also be considered if drugs are not effective.

5. Prognosis

Children with PME do poorly, while those with benign myoclonic epilepsy and juvenile myoclonic epilepsy do much better.

C. Myoclonic-Akinetic Epilepsy Syndrome

See Chapter 5.

VI. SITUATION-RELATED EPILEPSIES

A. Febrile Convulsions

B. Seizures with Special Modes of Precipitation

See Chapter 8.

VII. SPECIAL SYNDROMES

A. Landau-Kleffner Syndrome

1. Definition and Clinical Features

The Landau-Kleffner syndrome (LKS) is a rare childhood disorder consisting of an acquired aphasia and epileptiform discharges involving the temporal or parietal regions of the brain.

While there is a considerable amount of variation in the disorder, the typical history is that a child develops an abrupt or gradual loss of language ability and inattentiveness to sound, with onset during the first decade of life. This interruption in communication skills is generally closely preceded, accompanied, or followed by the onset of seizures or an abnormal EEG, or both. Receptive dysfunction, often referred to as auditory agnosia, may be the dominant feature early in the course of the disorder. In some children, the disorder progresses to the point where the child cannot even recognize sounds. In addition to the aphasia, many of the children have behavioral and psychomotor disturbances, often appearing autistic. The neurologic examination, other than the mental status examination, is usually normal.

The clinical course of LKS is variable with the long-term outcome of the aphasia quite unpredictable, despite the fact that epilepsy and EEG abnormalities frequently regress or disappear over time. Some patients with the syndrome have an abnormal EEG but never develop seizures.

A condition related to LKS is *epilepsy with continuous spike-wave discharges during sleep (CSWDS)*, a condition characterized by continuous spikes and waves during sleep. The disorder has also been termed "electrical status epilepticus during sleep (ESES)." Spike and wave activity is the dominant sleep pattern during sleep, occupying no less than 85% of the total slow-wave sleep time. The disorder begins during early childhood, peaking between 4 and 5 years of age. The children may have partial, generalized tonic-clonic, or myoclonic seizures. Seizures may occur during sleep or the awake state.

There are significant similarities between LKS and CSWDS, suggesting that the two disorders are part of the spectrum of seizure-related aphasia. Both disorders are associated with cognitive impairment, particularly language, and behavioral disturbances.

2. EEG Phenomena

There is not a specific EEG pattern in LKS. Most commonly there are repetitive spikes, sharp waves, and spike-and-wave activity in the temporal region or parietal-occipital regions, bilaterally. Sleep usually activates the record and, at times, the abnormality is seen only in sleep recordings. The distinguishing feature of CSWDS is the continuous bilateral and diffuse slow spike-wave persisting through all of the slow sleep stages. The spike-wave index (total minutes of all spike-waves x 100 divided by the total minutes of non-REM sleep without spike-wave) ranges from 85% to 100%.

3. Basic Mechanisms

While the pathogenesis of the language disorder in these patients is not known, it is possible that the epileptiform activity noted on the EEG results in "sub-clinical" seizures. Speech deficits may be explained on the basis of either disruption of normal connections or an excessive inhibitory reaction to epileptiform discharges. Speech usually does not improve in the syndrome unless there is improvement of the EEG. However, if the aphasia is simply the result of ongoing epileptiform activity, it seems strange that most antiepileptic drugs are ineffective. Furthermore, the severity of the aphasia does not always have a close correlation with the degree of EEG abnormality or clinical seizures.

Another viewpoint is that the epileptiform activity is an epiphenomenon and simply is reflective of an underlying cortical abnormality. Even if the EEG parallels speech recovery, this does not prove that epileptiform activity causes aphasia. It is possible that the decreased epileptiform activity during speech recovery simply reflects resolving injury to the speech areas.

4. Etiology

Neuroradiologic examinations are usually normal in LKS and, in most cases, the paroxysmal discharges recorded during wakefulness and sleep do not seem to be promoted by a detectable structural epileptogenic lesion. However, there have been a handful of cases of patients with the syndrome who have had tumors, neurocysticercosis, vasculitis, and encephalitis.

5. Treatment

Treatment of LKS and CSWDS can be frustrating. Unless there is objective evidence of changes in speech from an impartial, blinded observer, it is difficult to separate a placebo effect from drug-related improvement. While standard drugs may be helpful in reducing seizure frequency, there is usually not a significant improvement in language and cognitive function with these drugs. Corticosteroids resulted in improved speech, suppression of seizures, and normalization of the EEG in several small series of children. There is not enough experience with corticosteroid treatment to provide strict treatment guidelines. The authors usually treat children with LKS and CSWDS with 2 to 3 mg/kg/day of prednisone for 2 months. At that time, the prednisone is slowly tapered until the child is on 0.5 mg/kg every other day. If corticosteroids have been beneficial this dosage is usually maintained for 6 to 8 months. If treatment has not been effective the drug is discontinued. In cases of relapse the dosage is increased and maintained for a longer period of time.

Subpial cortical transections have been reported to be useful in patients with LKS. Unfortunately, as with steroids, this procedure has not been studied in any controlled manner.

6. Prognosis

The outcome in both LKS and CSWDS is variable. Recovery of language in LKS is highly dependent on age of onset of the syndrome, with the best recovery seen in children with early onset. Likewise, in CSWDS, outcome varies from full recovery to continued speech and cognitive impairment. Fortunately, most patients with CSWDS have some amelioration in their cognition and behavior over time.

REFERENCES

1. Berkovic SF, Andermann F, Carpenter S, Wolfe LS. Progressive myoclonus epilepsies: specific causes and diagnosis. *N Engl J Med* 1986;315:296–305.

2. Berkovic SF, So NK, Andermann F. Progressive myoclonus epilepsies: clinical and neurophysiological diagnosis. *J Clin Neurophysiol* 1991;8:261–274.
3. Engel J, Pedley TA, eds. *Epilepsy: a comprehensive textbook.* Philadelphia: Lippincott–Raven, 1997. Chaps. 51–54, 216–219, 220–228.
4. Ferrie CD, Beaumanois A, Geurin R, et al. Early onset benign occipital seizure susceptibility syndrome. *Epilepsia* 1997;38:285–293.
5. Gastaut H. Benign epilepsy of childhood with occipital paroxysms. In: Roger J, Bureau M, Dravet C, Dreifuss FE, Perret A, Wolf P, eds. *Epileptic syndromes in infancy, childhood and adolescence.* 2nd ed. London: John Libbey;1992:201–217.
6. Gabbi G, Gueirini R. Childhood epilepsy with occipital spikes and other benign localization-related epilepsies. In: Engel J, Pedley TA, eds. *Epilepsy: a comprehensive textbook.* Philadelphia: Lippincott–Raven, 1997.
7. Holmes GL. Rolandic epilepsy: clinical and electroencephalographic features. In: Degen R, Dreifuss FE, eds. *Benign localized and generalized epilepsies of early childhood.* Amsterdam: Elsevier Science Publishers B.V. 1992:29–43.
8. Holmes GL, McKeever M, Adamson M. Absence seizures in children: clinical and electroencephalographic features. *Ann Neurol* 1987;21:268–273.
9. Janz D. The idiopathic generalized epilepsies of adolescence with childhood and juvenile age of onset. *Epilepsia* 1997;38:4–11.
10. Landau WM, Kleffner FR. Syndrome of acquired aphasia with convulsive disorder in children. *Neurology* 1957;7:523–530.
11. Lerman P. Benign childhood epilepsy with centrotemporal spikes. In: Engel J, Pedley TA, eds. *Epilepsy: A comprehensive textbook.* Philadelphia: Lippincott–Raven, 1997.
12. Loiseau P, Pestre M, Dartigues JF, Commenges D, Barberger-Gateau C, Cohadon S. Long-term prognosis in two forms of childhood epilepsy: typical absence seizures and epilepsy with rolandic (centrotemporal) EEG foci. *Ann Neurol* 1983;13:642–648.
13. Lombroso C. Sylvian seizures and midtemporal spike foci in children. *Arch Neurol* 1967;17:52–59.
14. Markand ON. Slow spike-wave activity in EEG and associated clinical features: often called 'Lennox' or

'Lennox-Gastaut' syndrome. *Neurology* 1977;27: 746–757.

15. Montovani JF, Landau WM. Acquired aphasia with convulsive disorder: course and prognosis. *Neurology* 1980;30:524–529.

16. Panayiotopoulos CP. Benign childhood epilepsy with occipital paroxysms: a 15-year prospective study. *Ann Neurol* 1989;26:51–56.

17. Pearl PL, Holmes GL. Absence seizures. In: Dodson WE, Pellock JM, eds. *Pediatric epilepsy: diagnosis and therapy*. New York: Demos Publication;1993:157–169.

18. Penry JK, Porter RJ, Dreifuss FE. Simultaneous recording of absence seizures with videotape and electroencephalography. *Brain* 1975;98:427–440.

19. Prasad AN, Stafstrom CE, Holmes GL. Alternative epilepsy therapies: the ketogenic diet, immunoglobulins, and steroids. *Epilepsia* 1996;37(Suppl. 1):581–595.

20. Pravet C, Genton P. Lennox-Gastaut syndrome and other childhood epileptic encephalopathies. In: Engel J, Pedley TA, eds. *Epilepsy: a comprehensive textook*. Philadelphia: Lippincott–Raven, 1997.

21. Sato S, Dreifuss FE, Penry JK. Prognostic factors in absence seizures. *Neurology* 1976;26:788–796.

22. Sato S, Dreifuss FE, Penry JK, et al. Long-term follow-up of absence seizures. *Neurology* 1983;33:1590–1595.

23. Sato S, White BG, Penry JK, et al. Valproic acid versus ethosuximide in the treatment of absence seizures. *Neurology* 1982;32:157–163.

24. Smith M. Landau–Kleffner syndrome. In: Engel J, Pedley TA, eds. *Epilepsy: a comprehensive textook*. Philadelphia: Lippincott–Raven, 1997.

25. So NK, Anderman F. Rasmussen's syndrome. In: Engel J, Pedley TA, eds. *Epilepsy: a comprehensive textook*. Philadelphia: Lippincott–Raven, 1997.

26. Wirrell EC, Camfield PR, Camfield CS, Dooley JM, Gordon KE. Accidental injury is a serious risk in children with typical absence seizures. *Arch Neurol* 1996; 53:929–932.

27. Wirrell EC, Camfield CS, Camfield PR, Gordon KE, Dooley JM. Long-term prognosis of childhood absence epilepsy: regression or progression to juvenile myoclonic epilepsy. *Neurology* 1996;47:912–918.

28. Wyllie E, ed. *The treatment of epilepsy: principles and practice,* 2nd ed. Baltimore: Williams and Wilkins, 1997, Chaps. 29–37, 41.

EPILEPSIES WITH JUVENILE AND ADULT ONSET (12 YEARS AND OLDER)

TABLE 1. Epilepsies and epilepsy syndromes with juvenile and adult onset (12 years and older)

I. Localization-related/symptomic epilepsies
  A. Temporal lobe epilepsy syndromes (SPS, CPS, TCS)
  B. Frontal lobe epilepsy syndromes (SPS, CPS, TCS)
  C. Parietal lobe epilepsy syndromes (SPS, CPS, TCS)
  D. Occipital lobe epilepsy syndromes (SPS, CPS, TCS)
II. Generalized/idiopathic epilepsies
  A. Juvenile absence epilepsy (ABS, TCS)
  B. Juvenile myoclonic epilepsy (MYO, TCS, ABS)
  C. Epilepsy with tonic-clonic seizures on awakening (TCS)
  D. Epilepsy with random tonic-clonic seizures (TCS)
III. Generalized/either idiopathic or symptomatic
  A. Progressive myoclonic seizures (MYO)
IV. Situation-related epilepsies
  A. Alcohol/drug related (TCS)
  B. Eclampsia (TCS)
  C. Seizures with special modes of precipitation
      (SPS, CPS, TCS, MYO, ABS)

ABS = absence seizures; CLO = clonic seizures; CPS = complex partial (psychomotor, temporal lobe) seizures; MYO = myoclonic seizures; SPS = simple partial (focal) seizures; TCS = tonic-clonic (grand mal) seizures.

The epilepsies and epilepsy syndromes with juvenile and adult onset (12 years and older) and accompanying seizure type are listed in Table 7-1. This table serves as an outline of this chapter.

I. LOCALIZATION-RELATED/SYMPTOMATIC EPILEPSIES

Localization-related/symptomatic epilepsies can occur at any age. Three seizure types occur with these epilepsies: simple partial (focal), complex partial (psychomotor, temporal lobe) and tonic-clonic (grand mal). The clinical and EEG features of these three seizure types are reviewed in Chapter 2; management and prognosis are reviewed in Chapter 3. Differential diagnostic entities to consider in children and adults when diagnosing these seizure types are listed in Chapter 3 and reviewed in Chapter 9.

Depending on locus of onset, four groups of localization-related/symptomatic epilepsy syndromes have been recognized (Table 7-1). Clinical and EEG features, and management and prognosis of these four syndromes are reviewed in Chapter 3.

II. GENERALIZED/IDIOPATHIC EPILEPSIES

A. Juvenile Absence Epilepsy

Childhood and juvenile absence epilepsy are reviewed in detail with childhood epilepsies in Chapter 6. Only special features of this epilepsy in adults will be presented here.

Childhood and juvenile-onset absence epilepsy persist into adulthood in 30% to 50% of patients and may be difficult to control. Absence seizures may be overlooked during childhood and first come to medical attention in the late teens or early 20s (e.g., after joining the military, going to college, or starting a job). Absence seizures must be clearly differentiated from complex partial seizures, because both may present with lapses of consciousness and automatisms (see Chapter 9). The treatment is different for both seizure types. Hyperventilation is useful for producing clinical and EEG manifestations of absence seizures in patients of all ages.

Absence seizures may be difficult to control in adults who fail to "outgrow" absence seizures. The combination of ethosuximide and valproic acid is sometimes effective when monotherapy fails.

Approximately one-third to one-half of patients with absence seizures will experience tonic-clonic seizures at some time during their lives. Unlike absence seizures, tonic-clonic seizures persist past the teens in the majority of patients.

Absence status epilepticus is more common in adults than in children. Clinical, EEG, and management aspects of absence status epilepticus are described in Chapter 12.

B. Juvenile Myoclonic Epilepsy

1. Definition and Clinical Features

Juvenile myoclonic epilepsy (JME) is a syndrome of myoclonic and tonic-clonic seizures with typical onset at 12–18 years (range 8–30 years) of age. It is the most common cause of primarily generalized myoclonic and tonic-clonic seizures in adults. Other synonyms for this syndrome are "impulsive petit mal" and "Syndrome of Janz."

The characteristic symptom is sudden mild-to-moderate jerks of the shoulders and arms that occur shortly after awakening. No disturbance of consciousness is noticeable. Jerks also may occur when falling asleep or at any time. Approximately 90% of patients also have tonic-clonic seizures, which also tend to occur shortly after awakening in the morning. In approximately one-half of patients, the myoclonic seizures precede the tonic-clonic seizures and vice versa. Ten to thirty percent of patients also have absence seizures. The absence seizures usually begin before the other seizure types and are relatively infrequent, brief, and not associated with myoclonic jerks or automatisms. Juvenile myoclonic epilepsy is a genetically determined syndrome (short arm of chromosome 6, JME-1 locus) whose molecular defect remains unidentified.

2. EEG Features

Interictal EEGs in untreated persons show bilateral, symmetric, synchronous, and diffuse polyspike- and slow-wave complexes with a frequency of 4 to 6 Hz. During myoclonias, 6 to 16 Hz polyspikes lead to higher voltage-recruiting patterns at the start of tonic-clonic seizures. There is no close phase correlation between EEG spikes and jerks. During absence seizures the 4 to 6 Hz discharges may slow to 3 Hz and occur as polyspike-wave or spike wave. Frequently, patients are photosensitive.

3. Diagnosis

A history of myoclonic and/or tonic-clonic seizures on awakening suggests the diagnosis. The myoclonic and absence seizures are often ignored by the patient, and the physician should always inquire regarding myoclonic seizures on awakening and absence seizures in a teenager or young adult presenting with tonic-clonic seizures. The family history is positive for seizures in one-half of patients. The diagnosis is confirmed by EEG. Intelligence is in the normal range. Neurologic examination and imaging studies are normal.

4. Differential Diagnosis

Juvenile myoclonic epilepsy must be differentiated from other myoclonic epilepsies of childhood, progressive myoclonic epilepsies, epilepsy with grand mal seizures on awakening, epilepsy with random tonic-clonic seizures, and juvenile absence epilepsy. Note that in JME, myoclonic seizures, absence seizures, and tonic-clonic seizures on awakening can occur in the same patient at different times.

There are a number of rare myoclonic epilepsies which occur earlier in life than JME: myoclonic absence, myoclonic-astatic, early childhood myoclonic epilepsy, and benign or severe myoclonic epilepsy in infants [see Chapters 5 and 6 and ref. (10)].

There are a number of rare, progressive myoclonic epilepsy syndromes in adults characterized by progressive neurologic deterioration, dementia, and ataxia (see Chapter 6); JME has none of these characteristics.

Epilepsy with grand mal seizures on awakening is closely related to JME (see following), but myoclonic and absence seizures are not present. In epilepsy with random tonic-clonic seizures, the tonic-clonic seizures occur at times other than on awakening, and myoclonic and absence seizures are absent.

In juvenile absence epilepsy myoclonic seizures are absent, and the tonic-clonic seizures occur randomly (i.e., not just upon awakening). The interictal-EEG findings of juvenile absence epilepsy (3 Hz spike-wave, usually exacerbated by hyperventilation, seldom photosensitive) are different from those in JME (4-6 Hz polyspike-wave, seldom exacerbated by hyperventilation, often photosensitive).

5. Management

Patients should be warned to avoid certain circumstances which can precipitate JME: sleep deprivation, early awakening, alcohol intake, fatigue, and flickering lights (in some patients). Valproic acid alone usually is effective in controlling all three seizure types in JME. When additional seizure control is needed, phenytoin is effective for the tonic-clonic seizures of JME; ethosuximide is effective for the absence seizures; clonazepam is effective for the myoclonic seizures. Carbamazepine is effective for the tonic-clonic seizures, but may make absence seizures worse. Uncontrolled studies suggest lamotrigine may be effective for all three seizure types (not FDA-approved indications). Dosing directions for the drugs in children and adults are given in Chapter 11, Tables 11-1 and 11-2.

6. Prognosis

The seizures usually can be completely controlled with medication. Unfortunately, JME tends to be a lifelong trait, and drugs seldom can be withdrawn without recurrence of seizures.

C. Epilepsy with Tonic-Clonic Seizures on Awakening

This is a syndrome similar to JME, with onset occurring mostly during the second decade of life. The tonic-clonic seizures occur exclusively or predominantly (>90% of the time) after awakening, regardless of the time of day, or in a second-seizure peak in the evening period of relaxation. Myoclonic and absence seizures do not occur. As with JME, a genetic predisposition has been noted, and there is evidence both epilepsies are linked to the JME-1 locus of chromosome 6. The EEG shows generalized spike-wave patterns and may show photosensitivity. The tonic-clonic seizures respond to valproic acid, phenytoin, or carbamazepine administered as directed in Chapter 11, Tables 11-2 (children) or 11-3 (adults).

D. Epilepsy with Random Tonic-Clonic Seizures

This syndrome also has onset during the second decade. Myoclonic or absence seizures are not present. Tonic-clonic seizures may occur any time (not just after awakening). There is a familial tendency for this disorder, but it is not linked to the JME-1 locus of chromosome 6. The seizures respond to valproic acid, phenytoin, or carbamazepine as directed in Chapter 11, Tables 11-2 (children) and 11-3 (adults).

III. GENERALIZED/EITHER IDIOPATHIC OR SYMPTOMATIC

A. Progressive Myoclonic Seizures (MYO, TLS, CLO)

See Chapter 6.

IV. SITUATION-RELATED EPILEPSIES

A. Alcohol/Drug Related (TCS)

B. Eclampsia (TCS)

C. Seizures with Special Modes of Precipitation (SPS, CPS, TCS, MYO, ABS)

See Chapter 8.

REFERENCES

1. Annegers JF. The epidemiology of epilepsy. In: Wyllie E, ed. *The treatment of epilepsy: principles and practice*, 2nd ed. Baltimore: Williams and Wilkins, 1997.

2. Browne TR, Feldman RG, eds. *Epilepsy: diagnosis and management*. Boston: Little Brown, 1983. (Contains series of reviews of epileptic seizures.)

3. Commission on Classification and Terminology of the International League Against Epilepsy. Proposal for revised clinical and electroencephalographic classification of epileptic seizures. *Epilepsia* 1981;22:489–501.

4. Commission on Classification and Terminology of the International League Against Epilepsy. Proposal for revised classification of epilepsies and epileptic syndromes. *Epilepsia* 1989;30:389–399.

5. Delgado-Escuto AV, Serratosa JM, Medina MT. Myoclonic seizures and progressive myoclonic epilepsy syndrome. In: Wyllie E, ed. *The treatment of epilepsy: principles and practice*. Baltimore: Williams and Wilkins, 1997.

6. Engel J, Pedley TA, eds. *Epilepsy: a comprehensive textbook*. Philadelphia: Lippincott–Raven, 1997, Chaps. 51, 52, 220–228.

7. Gastaut H. Generalized convulsive seizures without local onset. In: Vinken PJ, Bruyn GW, eds. *Handbook at clinical neurology*. Vol 15, The Epilepsies. Amsterdam: Elsevier, 1974.

8. Greenburg DA, Dufner M, Resor S, et al. The genetics of generalized epilepsies of adolescent onset: differences between juvenile myoclonic epilepsy and epilepsy with random grand mal and with awakening grand mal. *Neurology* 1995;45:942–946.

9. Hauser WA. The natural history of seizures. In: Wyllie E, ed. *The treatment of epilepsy: principles and practice*, 2nd ed. Baltimore: Williams and Wilkins, 1997.

10. Janz D. The idiopathic generalized epilepsies of adolescence with childhood and juvenile age of onset. *Epilepsia* 1997;39:4–11.

11. Mattson RH. Selection of antiepileptic drugs. In: Levy RH, Mattson RH, Meldrum BS, eds. *Antiepileptic drugs*, 4th ed. New York: Raven Press, 1995.

12. Serratosa JM, Delgado-Escueto AV. Juvenile myoclonic epilepsy. In: Wyllie E, ed. *The treatment of epilepsy: principles and practice*, 2nd ed. Baltimore: Williams and Wilkins, 1997.

13. Wyllie E, ed. *The treatment of epilepsy: principles and practice,* 2nd ed. Baltimore: Williams and Wilkins, 1997, Chaps. 11, 12, 30–34.

SITUATION-RELATED EPILEPSIES

TABLE 8-1. Situation-related epilepsies and accompanying seizure types

I. Febrile convulsions (TCS, TON)
II. Alcohol-related (TCS)
III. Drug-related (TCS)
IV. Eclampsia (TCS)
V. Seizures with specific modes of precipitation: reflex epilepsies (SPS, CPS, TCS, MYO, ABS)

ABS = absence seizures; CPS = complex partial (psychomotor, temporal lobe) seizures; MYO = myoclonic seizures; SPS = simple partial (focal) seizures; TCS = tonic-clonic (grand mal) seizures; TON = tonic seizures.

The situation related epilepsies and their accompanying seizure types are listed in Table 8-1. This table also serves as an outline of this chapter.

I. FEBRILE SEIZURES
A. Definition
A febrile seizure is a seizure disorder that occurs in children between 6 months and 5 years of age, in association with a fever but without evidence of intracranial infection. The first febrile seizure in the majority of children occurs before 3 years, with the average age of onset between 18 and 22 months. Most studies have demonstrated a higher incidence in boys.

B. Seizure Phenomena
Febrile seizures may be of any type, although they are usually generalized tonic-clonic or tonic in type. Febrile seizures are classified as complex if the seizure duration is greater than 15 min, there is more than 1 seizure in 24 hr, or focal features are present.

C. EEG Phenomena
The EEG has not been found to be useful in the evaluation of a child with febrile seizures. While there remains some controversy, most authorities feel that the EEG is a poor predictor of either febrile or afebrile seizure recurrence. Approximately one-third of patients with febrile seizures will have an abnormal EEG when the record is obtained within a week of the seizure. While the most

common abnormality is occipital slowing, generalized spike-and-wave and focal spikes may occur. However, this epileptiform activity is not predictive of the eventual development of epilepsy. The authors do not recommend the use of routine EEG in patients with febrile seizures.

D. Management

The physician must first identify whether there is an underlying illness that requires immediate, specific treatment. The most urgent diagnostic decision is whether to do a lumbar puncture. One of the earliest signs of meningitis may be a seizure, which like a febrile seizure, is usually short and generalized tonic-clonic in type. While meningitis typically results in meningismus, in patients under the age of 2 years clinical signs of meningitis may be minimal or absent.

In the absence of specific clinical indications, there is little evidence in the literature indicating that other tests are helpful in determining etiology of seizures associated with fever. Skull films, serum glucose, calcium, blood urea nitrogen (BUN), and electrolytes are of low-yield and are not routinely recommended. Brief, single, self-limited febrile seizures from which the child fully recovers are seldom caused by conditions such as hypoglycemia or toxins. Unless the physical examination points to a possible structural lesion, a computed tomography (CT) or magnetic resonance imaging (MRI) scan is not warranted in the evaluation of febrile seizures. Since the EEG is of questionable value following febrile seizures, routine EEGs are not necessary.

E. Treatment

There has been a marked change in the management of febrile seizures over the past decade. The recent trend has been away from treating all children with febrile seizures with long-term antiepileptic drugs. This change in attitude has arisen primarily because of the results of large epidemiologic studies demonstrating that the prognosis for febrile seizures is excellent.

Phenobarbital and primidone have been the mainstays of prophylactic treatment of febrile seizures. However, a study by Farwell and colleagues (3) has raised questions about this approach. In this prospective study, 217 children between 8 and 36 months of age who had at least one febrile seizure and were at heightened risk for further seizures (an age of less than 12 months; a seizure that lasted more than 15 min, was focal, or recurred within 24 hr; nonfebrile seizures in a parent or sibling; or abnormal neurologic status before the index seizure), were randomized to phenobarbital or placebo treatment. The authors found that phenobarbital was not statistically more effective than placebo in preventing seizure recurrence. In addition, after 2 years the mean intelligence quotient (IQ) was 8.4 points lower in the group assigned to phenobarbital, than in the placebo group. Six months later, after the medication had been tapered and discontinued, the mean IQ was still 5.2 points lower in the phenobarbital-treated group. The investigators analyzed results by intention to treat (i.e., all treated patients counted), as opposed to examining IQ, and recurrence risk in children who actually had therapeutic levels of phenobarbital. It is also uncertain whether the IQ differences will be persistent. Nevertheless, the study does suggest that phenobarbital treatment may be more harmful than helpful in the treatment of febrile seizures.

Rectal and oral diazepam administered at the time of a febrile illness have been shown to be effective in the prevention of febrile seizure recurrences. It is likely that this approach will supplant the use of chronic phenobarbital therapy.

F. Prognosis

Febrile seizures are associated with a very low mortality rate. When deaths do occur, they are usually secondary to the agent causing the fever or an antecedent neurologic disorder. In addition, there is a low incidence of acquired motor or intellectual abnormalities following a febrile seizure.

While relatively few children who experience febrile seizures develop epilepsy, recurrences of febrile seizures are commonplace. In the National Collaborative Perinatal Project (NCPP), approximately one-third of the children had at least one recurrence, and one-half of those who had one recurrence had an additional attack.

Recurrence risk is not uniform for all children with febrile seizures. The most important factor appears to be age of onset of the first febrile seizure. The younger the child at the first attack, the more likely are further febrile seizures. Children who experience their first seizure when less than 13 months of age have greater than a 2:1 chance for developing further febrile seizures. This compares with a risk of approximately 20% in patients that have their first febrile seizure after age 32 months.

Three-fourths of recurrence takes place within 1 year of the first febrile seizure and 90% within 2 years.

While children who have one or more febrile seizures are at higher risk than the normal population for the development of epilepsy, the risk is quite small. In a large epidemiologic study in the United States, Nelson and Ellenberg (14,15) examined the frequency of afebrile seizures in 1,706 children who had experienced at least one febrile seizure and were followed to the age of 7 years. At least one afebrile seizure had occurred by the age of 7 in 3% of the patients with febrile seizures. Two percent of the group had two or more afebrile seizures by age 7, and would be considered to have epilepsy. Of 39,179 children who had never been reported to experience a febrile seizure, 0.5% had epilepsy by age 7. The risk for developing epilepsy was, therefore, 4 times higher in the group that had febrile seizures.

The risk for developing unprovoked seizures is increased by several factors. These include: neurodevelopmental anomalies, complex febrile seizures, recurrent febrile seizures, brief duration of fever before initial seizure, and family history of epilepsy.

Prolonged febrile seizures have been implicated as a predisposing factor for the development of temporal lobe epilepsy and mesial temporal sclerosis, a pathologic condition of hippocampal sclerosis and atrophy with loss of neurons in the CA1 region and the endfolium (CA3/CA4), but with relative sparing of the CA2 region (see Chapter 3). Loss of dentate hilar neurons (endfolium sclerosis) is a common feature, and in some patients may be the only apparent hippocampal lesion.

II. ALCOHOL-RELATED EPILEPSY SYNDROMES

A. Introduction

Most alcohol-related seizures are caused by alcohol withdrawal, and this condition will be reviewed in detail. However, one must be aware that alcoholics are at risk of having several other medical conditions which may present as seizures (see "Differential Diagnosis," Section II, E). One also must be aware that alcohol-withdrawal seizures frequently are accompanied by other symptoms and signs of alcohol withdrawal (anxiety, insomnia, irritability, nausea, tremor, tachycardia, hypertension, fever, hyperreflexia, and hallucinations), and may progress to delirium tremens. Alcoholism affects all social classes;

50% of alcoholics have attended college and hold managerial or professional positions.

B. Clinical Features of Alcohol-Withdrawal Seizures (Table 8-2)

Patients usually are chronic alcoholics 30 years of age or older. Ninety percent of alcohol-withdrawal seizures occur 7 to 48 hr after cessation of drinking, and 50% occur 13 to 24 hr after drinking has ceased. Thus, some alcohol often is still present in the plasma at the time of the seizure, and the patient may have the odor of alcohol on his breath when brought to the hospital. Alcohol-withdrawal seizures can occur up to 7 days after stopping drinking. Clinical examination frequently reveals tremulousness and some myoclonic jerks of the extremities. Seizures typically are generalized onset tonic-clonic in type. Seizures may be single (40%) or multiple (usually 2 to 4). The time between the first and last seizure usually is less than 6 hr. If untreated, one-third of patients will go on to develop full-blown delirium tremens, and a small number will develop tonic-clonic status epilepticus.

C. EEG Features of Alcohol-Withdrawal Seizures

The interictal EEG usually is normal, and the ictal EEG shows the typical findings of tonic-clonic seizures. In 50% of untreated patients there is heightened excitability to photic stimulation (photoconvulsive or photomyoclonic responses) for 12 to 130 hr after cessation of drinking. This can be a clue to surreptitious alcoholism in a patient presenting with a first tonic-clonic seizure. Photic excitability usually disappears immediately after treatment with a benzodiazepine.

D. Basic Mechanisms and Etiology

Alcohol dependence is considered divisible into two types: (a) *psychological dependence*, in which the rewarding effects of alcohol play a primary role; and (b) *chemical dependence*, in which adaptive changes in the brain initiate punishing effects on withdrawal of alcohol, and suppression of these becomes the primary motive for using the drug. The neurochemical basis for the rewarding effects of alcohol may be the potentiation of gamma-aminobutyric acid (GABA) at $GABA_A$ receptors (causing relaxation) and release of dopamine from mesolimbic neurones (causing euphoria). The adaptive changes which cause the alcohol-withdrawal syndrome are not known for certain. Habitua-

TABLE 8-2. Causes of seizures associated with alcohol use

Seizure category	Onset age	Acute intoxication	First 48 hr of withdrawal	Seizures after prolonged abstinence	Interictal EEG	Photic Sensitivity	Treatment
Acute seizures (electrolyte disturbance, hypoglycemia, meningitis)	Any age	Yes	Yes	No	Abnormal (slow)	Absent	Specific
Withdrawal seizures ("rum fits," alcoholic epilepsy)	30+ (90%)	No	Yes	No	90% normal	50% photo-myoclonic (photomyogenic) or photo-convulsive	Lorazepam or diazepam and abstinence
Epilepsy following alcoholism	Any age	Infrequently	Yes	Yes	Usually abnormal (epileptiform patterns or slowing)	50% photo-myoclonic (photomyo-genic) or photo-convulsive	Lorazepam or diazepam, maintenance anti-epileptic drugs, and abstinence

Modified from Mattson, RH. Seizures associated with alcohol use and alcohol withdrawal. In: Browne TR, Feldman RG, eds. *Epilepsy: diagnosis and management*. Boston: Little Brown, 1983, with permission.

tion in GABA$_A$ receptors, activation of NMDA receptors, elevated calcium flux at voltage-operated calcium channels, and increased release of central catecholamines all have been reported. Animal and clinical data suggest that repeated episodes of alcohol withdrawal may lead to an increase in severity of signs and symptoms on subsequent episodes of withdrawal, including greater risk of alcohol-withdrawal seizures ("kindling"). See the reviews of Littleton and Little (10) and McMicken and Freedland (13) for further details.

E. Differential Diagnosis

Alcohol-withdrawal seizures must be differentiated from other causes of seizures in patients with alcoholism (see Table 8-2) including: (a) withdrawal from sedative drugs (benzodiazepines, barbiturates); (b) drug intoxication (cocaine, amphetamines, phencyclidine); (c) head trauma (contusion, subdural hematoma, intracerebral hematoma); (d) stroke; (e) infections (meningitis, cerebral abscess); (f) metabolic (hypomagnesemia, hyponatremia, hypoglycemia); and (g) chronic, recurring epilepsy (may be exacerbated by alcohol withdrawal). Multiple causes may be present.

F. Management

1. Evaluation

A seizure history and an alcohol history should be obtained from the patient and from reliable observers. Patients must be evaluated for other causes of seizures (see earlier) and for complications of alcoholism, especially those which may precipitate abrupt alcohol withdrawal (meningitis, pneumonia, peritonitis, cranial or other trauma, gastrointenstinal bleeding, pancreatitis). Routine tests include complete blood count, chemical screen, toxic screen (for cocaine, barbiturates, and benzodiazepines), and chest x-ray. Any fever should be vigorously investigated. Unexplained fever may be caused by meningitis occurring without nuchal rigidity. Unexplained fever or fever with nuchal rigidity requires a lumbar puncture after increased intracranial pressure is excluded by CT or MRI scan. Such scans are also indicated if there is evidence of head trauma, a focally abnormal neurologic examination, or focal features to the seizures. EEG is discussed previously.

2. General Measures

a. Stabilize vital signs.
b. Immediately treat life-threatening conditions (status epilepticus, myocardial infarction).
c. Perform diagnostic evaluation (see earlier).
d. Thiamine 50 or 100 mg IM or IV to all patients **before** glucose is administered (administration of glucose before thiamine may deplete thiamine stores and precipitate Wernicke's disease). Multivitamins are of no proven value.
e. Correct fluid and electrolyte (Mg, K, Na) disturbances.

Note that excess fluid may elevate intracranial pressure in patients with mass lesions. Hyponatremia necessitates therapy only when symptomatic or severe; excessively rapid correction of sodium may precipitate central pontine myelinolysis. Hypomagnesemia may contribute to seizures or tremors; administer no more than 1 mg IV of MgS04 every 6 hours for patients with normal renal function.

3. Specific Measures

Lorazepam 2 to 5 mg IM or IV usually will stop alcohol-withdrawal seizures. Additional doses of 2 mg every 4 hr as needed by any route may be given to stop later withdrawal seizures (uncommon) or recurrence of other withdrawal symptoms (common).

Prolonged seizure activity can be treated with diazepam 2.5 mg/min until seizures stop (check for respiratory depression and/or hypotension). This can be followed with 5 to 10 mg doses every 4 to 8 hr as needed for later withdrawal seizures or recurrence of withdrawal symptoms.

The immediate and follow-up doses of benzodiazepines required to produce the desired state (no seizures, relaxed but awake) vary greatly. The initial dose should be the minimal dose which stops seizures and relieves withdrawal symptoms. Follow-up doses should be on an "as-needed" basis because lorazepam and diazepam can accumulate to toxic levels if given repeatedly. Phenytoin has no value for alcohol-withdrawal seizures, but may be of value for chronic epilepsy exacerbated by alcohol withdrawal. A loading dose of phenytoin may be given following procedures described in Chapter 7.

III. DRUG-RELATED EPILEPSY SYNDROMES

A. Recreational Drug-Induced Seizures

Amphetamines, cocaine, phencyclidine and combinations of these drugs are the most common causes of recreational drug-induced seizures. Seizures are independent of route of administration and may occur in first-time or chronic abusers.

1. Amphetamines, Cocaine, and Phencyclidine

A. INTRODUCTION AND MECHANISMS OF ACTION. *Amphetamines* include amphetamine sulfate (Benzedrine), dextroamphetamine (Dexedrine), and methamphetamine (Methedrine, "ice"). Amphetamines are sympathetic stimulants that act through norepinephrine- and dopamine-mediated systems. Amphetamines may be smoked or taken orally.

Cocaine is a powerful sympathetic and central nervous system (CNS) stimulant and an effective local anesthetic. The sympathomimetic effects result from blocking the reuptake of the neurotransmitters norepinephrine, acetylcholine, serotonin, and dopamine by presynaptic neurones. Cocaine may be smoked ("crack") or taken by nasal, oral, or intravenous routes. Cocaine frequently is "cut" with other drugs of abuse (amphetamines, opiates, phencyclidine).

Phencyclidine ("PCP," "angel dust") is a powerful sympathetic stimulant and psychotomimetic that may produce CNS stimulation or depression, depending upon dosage. At high doses it also has cholinergic properties. Phencyclidine may be smoked or taken by the nasal, oral, or intravenous routes.

B. CLINICAL FEATURES. All three drugs have many similarities in clinical features and treatment because all three are sympathetic stimulants that also can cause CNS stimulation.

Minor toxic manifestations include: tachypnea, tachycardia (occasionally, bradycardia with cocaine), mild hypertension, dry mouth, dizziness, chest pains, palpitations, abdominal cramps, nausea, diarrhea, mydriasis, diaphoresis, flushing, hyperactivity, hyperreflexia, irritability, confusion, apprehension, and hallucinations.

Major toxic manifestations include: severe hypertension (may be associated with intracranial hemorrhage), tachyarrhythmias (may progress to ventricular tachycardia or fibrillation), severe hyperthermia (may lead to coagulopathies, rhabdomyolysis, or renal failure), seizures (tonic-clonic), acidosis, delirium, psychosis, coma, and myocardial ischemia or infarction. Hypotension or circulatory collapse (sometimes fatal) may occur because of cardiac arrhythmias, myocardial infarction, or catecholamine depletion.

Special features of *cocaine* intoxication include respiratory depression (often preceded by a tonic-clonic seizure, may lead to sudden death) and prominent cardiac toxicity (sensitizes the myocardium to epinephrine and norepinephrine, direct cardiotoxic effect, and causes coronary artery spasm).

Special features of *phencyclidine* intoxication include the triad of altered mental status (agitation, confusion, violent or bizarre behavior, psychosis, catatonia, stupor, coma), hypertension, and horizontal or vertical nystagmus. Bronchial hypersecretion, bronchospasm, or dystonic reactions also may occur.

C. MANAGEMENT. *Seizures* are managed acutely with intravenous lorazepam or diazepam. Adequate doses should be administered to terminate seizures and to diminish agitation, reduce hypertension, and slow tachycardia. Repetitive or prolonged seizures require the administration of a loading dose of phenobarbital or phenytoin following procedures described in Chapter 7. General anesthesia with pentobarbital may be necessary in persistent seizures. Patients with seizures should be evaluated for intracranial hemorrhage or other new CNS lesions, and for rhabdomyolysis.

Other aspects of management include provision of a cool and quiet environment, gastric decontamination, sedation, and treatment of other manifestations including arrhythmias, hypertension, hypotension, respiratory depression, hyperthermia, chest pain, behavioral disturbances, uncontrollable motor activity and (for phencyclidine) dystonic reactions and bronchospasm. For these topics the reader is referred to a textbook of emergency medicine such as Stein and Chudnofsky (19).

2. Opiates

Although opiates generally cause CNS depression, overdosage with meperidine (Demerol) or propoxyphene (Talwin) may cause seizures. Naloxone hydrochloride is used to reverse the CNS effects (including seizures) of opiate intoxication. Propoxyphene overdosage may require larger than average doses.

B. Nonrecreational Drug-Induced Seizures

A long list of drugs prescribed for valid indications may precipitate seizures (Table 8-3).

Antidepressants and antipsychotics draw special consideration because of the not infrequent association of epilepsy with depression or psychosis. In general, the risk of seizures is small (a few percent or less) and the risk of depression or psychosis is great. Therefore, most experts in epilepsy permit full therapeutic dosages of antidepressant or antipsychotic medication in patients with epilepsy and significant depression or psychosis. Imipramine has a seizure rate of 0.3% to 0.6% at effective doses. The rate is probably lower for desipramine, fluoxetine, sertraline, flavoxamine, trazodone, nomifensine, and monoamine oxidase inhibitors [see reviews of Gilmore (8) and

TABLE 8-3. Drugs reported to precipitate seizures

Anticholinesterases	Nalidixic acid
Antidepressants	
Antihistamines	Narcotics
Antipsychotics	
Aqueous iodinated contrast agents	
	Oxytocin
Baclofen	
Beta blockers	Penicillins (especially, high dose)
	Phenothiazines
Chlorambucil	Procaine
Clozapine	
Cycloserine	Sympathomimetic agents
Ergonovine	Theophylline
	Tricyclics
Folic acid	
Foscarnet	
Haloperidol	
Imipenem	
Isoniazid	
Lidocaine	
Local anesthetics	
Mefenamic acid	
Methotrexate	
Metroridazol	
Misonidazole	

Modified from Gilmore RL. Seizures associated with nonneurological medical conditions. In: Wyllie E, ed. *The treatment of epilepsy: principles and practice*, 2nd ed. Baltimore: Williams and Wilkins, 1997, with permission.

Rosenstein et al. (22)]. Haloperidol may have a lower risk of precipitating seizures than phenothiazines.

High-dose intravenous penicillin may induce refractory status epilepticus, especially in patients with structural brain lesions. In this situation, the penicillin should be stopped immediately. Because of opposing actions on chloride channels, there is theoretical and empiric evidence phenobarbital reverses penicillin-induced seizures.

C. Sedative-Hypnotic Drug Withdrawal Seizures

1. Introduction and Mechanism of Action

The usual drugs causing withdrawal seizures are the sedative-hypnotic classes of drugs: barbiturates, benzodiazepines, and nonbarbiturate sedative-hypnotic agents. The mechanism of action and clinical features of these seizures are similar to alcohol-withdrawal seizures (see earlier).

2. Clinical Features

Onset of symptoms is dependent upon the duration of action and elimination half-life of the drug. Short-acting agents (e.g., alprazolam) may show withdrawal features within 24 hr; long-acting agents (e.g., diazepam, phenobarbital) may not show withdrawal features for 7 or more days. Symptoms include: weakness, insomnia, restlessness, anorexia, apprehension, headache, anxiety, and irritability. Signs include: tremor, fever, diaphoresis, dehydration, tachycardia, postural hypotension, dyspnea, and hyperreflexia. More serious findings include: myoclonus, seizures (may progress to status epilepticus), hyperpyrexia, hallucinations, and delirium.

3. Management

A. BARBITURATE OR NONBARBITURATE SEDATIVE-HYPNOTIC DEPENDENCY. Tolerance to sedative or hypnotic drugs is confirmed by administering 200 mg of pentobarbital IM or PO. Absence of sedation after 1 hour confirms tolerance. The patient's daily habitual dose is estimated by history. This dose of the abused drug (or an equivalent dose of phenobarbital up to 500 mg/day) is administered initially using a t.i.d. regimen and then gradually withdrawn. The following dosages are equivalent to 30 mg of phenobarbital: 100 mg pentobarbital, 500 mg chloral hydrate, 350 mg ethchlorvynol, 250 mg gluthimide, 250 mg methaqualone. See a textbook of emergency medicine such as Stein and Chudnofsky (19) for more details.

B. BENZODIAZEPINE DEPENDENCY. The patient is restarted on his or her daily dose of benzodiazepine (or an equivalent dose of phenobarbital up to 500 mg/d) using a t.i.d. regimen and then gradually withdrawn. The following dosages are equivalent to 30 mg of phenobarbital: 10 mg diazepam, 100 mg chlordiazepoxide.

D. Other Drug Withdrawal Seizures

Suddenly stopping opiates, amphetamines, or cocaine may induce tonic-clonic seizures. Suddenly stopping antiepileptic drug in a patient with epilepsy may precipitate seizures of the patient's usual type and/or status epilepticus.

E. Further Information

For further information readers are referred to their local poison centers, textbooks of medical emergencies [e.g., Stein and Chudnofsky (23)], or textbooks of toxicology [e.g., Goldfrank et al. (9)].

IV. ECLAMPSIA

A. Definition

Preeclampsia (toxemia gravidarum) is a pregnancy-induced disorder consisting of proteinuria and edema after the 20th week of gestation. The disorder is complex and may involve multiple organ systems with resultant pulmonary edema, oliguria, disseminated intravascular coagulopathy, and hepatic hemorrhages. Neurologic problems include headache, confusion, hyperreflexia, visual hallucinations, and even blindness. *Eclampsia* is the occurrence of convulsions, not caused by any coincidental neurologic disease such as long-standing epilepsy or intracranial structural lesions, in a woman who has the criteria for preeclampsia. The timing of seizures does not correlate with the severity of preeclampsia, and may occur even when there are few signs of preeclampsia.

The *causes* of preeclampsia-eclampsia are poorly understood, and it is not clear why seizures occur in the condition. There is evidence to suggest primary roles for endothelial damage, increased platelet aggregation and platelet consumption, as well as hypertension in the pathogenesis of the disorder. Pathologic examination of the brain has revealed diffuse cerebral edema, subarachnoid, subcortical, and petechial hemorrhages, and small infarctions of multiple areas in the brain.

B. Seizure Phenomena

The seizures may be partial or secondarily generalized. The seizures may appear before, during, or after childbirth. While they are most common within the first postpartum day, some patients may have them for as long as a month after delivery.

C. EEG Phenomena

EEGs are usually abnormal with focal or diffuse slowing and epileptiform activity. The epileptiform activity can be either focal, multifocal, or generalized in nature.

D. Treatment

Magnesium sulfate has been a standard treatment for treatment of both preeclampsia and eclampsia. Magnesium blocks the N-methyl-D-aspartate (NMDA) channel, a subtype of the glutamate receptor. It is possible, therefore, that magnesium blockade might work both as an anticonvulsant and neuroprotectant through this mechanism. Magnesium sulfate might also act as a calcium antaganist, preventing cerebral vasoconstriction, and subsequent epileptogenic cortical injury. While magnesium is not an effective treatment in other forms of epilepsy, its role in the treatment of seizures secondary to eclampsia has now been demonstrated. Unfortunately, magnesium sulfate is not without problems. It has a short half-life and can lead to sedation in the mother and hypotonia, hyporeflexia, and lethargy in the newborn.

Other drugs used in the treatment of seizures in eclampsia include phenytoin, diazepam, and chlormethiazole (not available in the United States). Phenytoin is particularly useful since it is effective in stopping the seizures and has minimal effects on the infant. As with status epilepticus, a loading dose of 15 mg/kg can be given with maintenance dosages started 12 hr later.

V. SEIZURES WITH SPECIFIC MODES OF PRECIPITATION (REFLEX EPILEPSIES)

In reflex epilepsy, seizures are regularly elicited by some specific stimulus or event. As commonly used, the reflex epilepsies include cases where the stimulus does not invariably produce a seizure and/or spontaneous seizures may occur.

Animal studies indicate reflex epilepsies may be caused by hyperexcitable neurones (on a structural or biochemical basis) in either primary receptive areas or their efferent connections. Entry of a stimulus activates these hyperexcitable neurons.

The types of stimuli which can evoke seizures are: visual (most common), complex activities, and proprioceptive.

A. Reflex Epilepsies with Visual Triggers

Visual reflex epilepsies are divided into two major groups, depending on whether seizures are induced by flickering light.

1. Seizures Induced by Flickering Light

These patients have tonic-clonic seizures (less often, absence or myoclonic) in response to flickering lights. Common precipitants include television (*television epilepsy*), video games, strobe lights, and light interrupted by trees and other objects while riding in a car. Seizures may occur only with photic stimulation or spontaneously in some patients. The seizures result in pleasurable sensations in some patients, resulting in self-induced flickering seizures. The resting EEG may show spike-wave discharges (especially with eye closure). Intermittent photic stimulation produces a photo-convulsive response in most patients. Typically, this group of seizures begins in the teens (female preponderance) and ends in the third decade.

2. Seizures not Induced by Flicker

Absence, myoclonus, or, more rarely, tonic-clonic seizures may occur in response to patterns (*pattern-sensitive seizures*). Patterns typically are striped and include common objects such as a television screen at short distances, striped clothing or drapes, or escalator steps. Eye closure may produce absence or myoclonic seizures in some persons (*seizures induced by eye closure*). Some persons with pattern-sensitive seizures or seizures induced by eye closure deliberately induce seizures because of pleasurable sensations associated with seizures.

B. Reflex Epilepsies Induced by Complex Activities

1. Seizures Induced by Thinking

These patients have myoclonic, absence or tonic-clonic seizures induced by specific thinking tasks. Such tasks include: card or board games, mental arithmetic, manipulation of spatial information, or making complex decisions. Often, there is more than one trigger and/or spontaneous seizures. Interictal EEGs are usually normal or show photosensitivity (25%). Ictal EEGs show generalized spike and wave patterns. Onset is in the teens with a male preponderance.

2. Musicogenic Epilepsy

These patients have simple and/or complex partial seizures in response to music (often, a specific piece). Emotional reactions mediated by limbic structures may play a role. Spontaneous seizures may also occur. Interictal EEGs show sharp and slow activity in temporal leads, more often on the right side.

3. Eating Epilepsy

Simple and/or complex partial seizures may be induced by the sight or smell of food or by gastric distention after eating food. Such patients usually have localization-related/symptomatic epilepsy originating in the temporolimbic area. Sensory, autonomic, or emotional inputs to this area during eating appear to activate seizures.

4. Reading Epilepsy and Language-Induced Epilepsy

Reading (usually prolonged), speaking, or writing may induce a typical seizure pattern of jaw jerks or clicks followed by a generalized convulsion if the inducing activity is not stopped. Absence of jaw jerks and/or presence of spontaneous seizures may occur. The interictal EEG usually is normal. Ictal EEGs may show focal (temporoparietal) or generalized discharges.

C. Reflex Epilepsies Induced by Proprioceptive Input (Movement-Induced Seizures)

Sudden, unexpected stimuli may produce lateralized tonic seizures in patients with lesions in the supplementary motor area or mesial frontal cortex (*startle epilepsy*). A second syndrome consists of attacks induced by active or passive movement without startle.

D. Management of Reflex Epilepsies

Management has three options: (a) avoidance of trigger, (b) desensitation therapy, (c) antiepileptic drugs. Avoidance of the trigger is effective in some, but not all, patients. Television epilepsy can be helped by increasing distance from the television, a small screen in a well-lit room, and use of a remote control to avoid need to approach the television closely. Desensitization therapy has been successfully applied to many forms of reflex epilepsy [see ref. (7)]. Valproic acid is the drug of choice for reflex epilepsies with absence, myoclonic, or tonic-clonic seizures. Partial seizures are treated with carbamazepine or phenytoin.

REFERENCES

1. Berg AT, Shinnar S. Unprovoked seizures in children with febrile seizures: short-term outcome. *Neurology* 1996;47:562–566.
2. Binnie CD. Simple reflex. In: Engel J, Pedley TA, eds. *Epilepsy: a comprehensive textbook*. Philadelphia: Lippincott–Raven, 1997.
3. Donaldson, JO. Eclampsia. In: Devinsky O, Feldmann E, Hainline B, eds. *Neurological complication of pregnancy*. New York: Raven Press, 1994.
4. Duchowny M. Febrile seizures in childhood. In: Wyllie E, ed. *The treatment of epilepsy: principles and practice, 2nd ed.* Baltimore: Williams and Wilkins, 1997.
5. Engel J, Pedley TA, eds. *Epilepsy: a comprehensive textbook.* Philadelphia: Lippincott–Raven, 1997, chapters 118, 230–240, 251.
6. Farwell JR, Lee YJ, Hirtz DG, et al., eds. Phenobarbital for febrile seizures—effects on intelligence and on seizure recurrence. *N Engl J Med* 1990;322:364–369.
7. Feldman RG, Ricks NL, Orren MM. Behavioral methods of seizure control. In: Browne TR, Feldman RG, eds. *Epilepsy: diagnosis and management.* Boston: Little Brown, 1983.
8. Gilmore RL. Seizures associated with nonneurological medical conditions. In: Wyllie E, ed. *The treatment of epilepsy: principles and practice*, 2nd ed. Baltimore: Williams and Wilkins, 1997.
9. Goldfrank LR, Flomenbaum NE, Lewin NA, et al., eds. *Toxicologic emergencies*. East Norwalk: Appleton & Lang, 1997.
10. Hirtz DG, Nelson KB. The natural history of febrile seizures. *Ann Rev Med* 1983;34:453–471.
11. Kaplan PW, Repke JT. Eclampsia. *Neurol Clin* 1994; 12:565–582.

12. Knudsen FU. Recurrence risk after first febrile seizure and effect of short term diazepam prophylaxis. *Arch Dis Child* 1985;60:1045–1049.

13. Leone M, Bottacchi E, Beghi E, et al. Alcohol use is a risk factor for a first generalized tonic-clonic seizure. *Neurology* 1997;48:614–620.

14. Littleton J, Little H. Current concepts of ethanol dependence. *Addiction* 1994;89:1397–1412.

15. Lucas MJ, Leveno KJ, Cunningham FG. A comparison of magnesium sulfate with phenytoin for prevention of eclampsia. *N Engl J Med* 1995;333:201–205.

16. Mattson, RH. Seizures associated with alcohol use and alcohol withdrawal. In: Browne TR, Feldman RG, eds. *Epilepsy: diagnosis and management.* Boston: Little Brown, 1983.

17. McMicken DB, Freedland ES. Alcohol-related seizures: pathophysiology, differential diagnosis, evaluation, and treatment. *Emerg Med Clin No Am* 1994; 14:1057–1079.

18. Nelson KB, Ellenberg JH. Predictors of epilepsy in children who have experienced febrile seizures. *N Engl J Med* 1976;295:1029–1033.

19. Nelson KB, Ellenberg JH. Prognosis in children with febrile seizures. *Pediatrics* 1978;61:720–727.

20. Porter RJ, Mattson RH. Alcohol and drug abuse. In: Engel J, Pedley TA, eds. *Epilepsy: a comprehensive textbook.* Philadelphia: Lippincott–Raven, 1997.

21. Roman NP, Colton T, Labazzo J, et al., eds. A controlled trial of diazepam administered during febrile illnesses to prevent recurrence of febrile seizures. *N Engl J Med* 1993;329:79–84.

22. Rosenstein DL, Nelson JC, Jacobs SC. Seizures associated with antidepressants: a review. *J Clin Psychiatry* 1993;54:289–299.

23. Stein RJ, Chudnofsky CR. *Emergency medicine.* Boston: Little, Brown, 1994.

24. Weiser HG, Hungerbuhler H, Siegel AM, et al. Musicogenic epilepsy: review of the literature and case report with single photon emission computed tomography. *Epilepsia* 1997;38:200–207.

25. Zifkin BG, Anderman F. Complex reflex epilepsies. In: Engel J, Pedley TA, eds. *Epilepsy: a comprehensive textbook.* Philadelphia: Lippincott–Raven, 1997.

DIAGNOSIS AND DIFFERENTIAL DIAGNOSIS

Diagnostic tasks in epilepsy management include establishing a seizure diagnosis and an etiologic diagnosis and identification of precipitating factors. This is accomplished by a combination of history taking, physical examination, electroencephalography, and laboratory examinations. Common differential diagnostic problems are reviewed at the end of this chapter.

I. SEIZURE DIAGNOSIS

The first step in managing a patient who may have epilepsy is establishing definitively whether or not the patient has epilepsy. If a patient who does not have epilepsy is given the diagnosis of epilepsy, he or she is unnecessarily subjected to many inconveniences, including medication that may produce serious side effects, expensive laboratory tests, loss of a driver's license, and possible loss of employment. Specific differential diagnostic entities, which must be differentiated from seizures, are discussed in the last section of this chapter.

If a patient has epilepsy, it is crucial to determine accurately which type(s) of epileptic seizure the patient has, in order that he or she be given correct therapy. The diagnosis of seizure type should be made according to the International Classification of Epileptic Seizures, reviewed briefly in Chapter 1 and in detail in Chapter 2.

II. ETIOLOGIC DIAGNOSIS

Epilepsy is a symptom, not a disease. A seizure can be a symptom of old or recent cerebral trauma, a brain tumor, a brain abscess, encephalitis, meningitis, a metabolic disturbance, drug intoxication, drug withdrawal, and many other disease processes. It is imperative that the underlying cause of a patient's seizure be identified and treated, so that a reversible cerebral disease process is not overlooked and seizure control can be facilitated.

III. PRECIPITATING FACTORS

In addition to determining the underlying cause(s) of a patient's seizure disorder, it is also important to identify and manage factors that precipitate seizures in a given individual, such as anxiety, sleep deprivation, and alcohol withdrawal (see Fig. 9-1). Management of such precipitating factors reduces seizure frequency as well as the patient's need for medication.

IV. HISTORY

The best way to diagnose which type of seizure a patient has is to actually observe a seizure, although the physician usually does not have the opportunity to do so. Often, the most important differential diagnostic information is contained in the history gathered from the patient, reliable observers, or both.

History for seizure diagnosis should include exact details of events before, during, and after the seizure obtained from the patient and observers. Partial seizure symptoms and signs (motor, sensory, autonomic, psychic), alteration of consciousness, automatisms, tonic and/or clonic movements, tongue biting, incontinence, and postictal behavior are important details. The duration, time of occurrence (e.g., upon awakening, when drowsy, during sleep), and frequency of seizures also are important. Past or current occurrence of other seizure types (especially myoclonic or absence) often is not volunteered by the patient and should be specifically asked for. Specific questions regarding entities which may be confused with seizures are discussed later in this chapter.

History for etiology should include questions regarding family history of epilepsy, head trauma, birth complications, febrile convulsions, middle ear infections and sinus infections (which may erode through bone and cause cerebral focus), alcohol or drug abuse, and symptoms of malignancy.

History for precipitating factors should include factors such as fever, anxiety, sleep deprivation, menstrual cycle, alcohol, hyperventilation, flickering lights, or television (see Fig. 9-1).

V. PHYSICAL EXAMINATION

The physical examination should be directed toward uncovering evidence of past or recent head trauma, infections of the ears and sinuses, congenital abnormalities (e.g., hemiatrophy, stigmata of tuberous sclerosis), focal or diffuse neurologic abnormalities, stigmata of alcohol or drug abuse, and signs of malignancy. Subtle but "hard" findings may be useful in uncovering evidence of focal brain dysfunction indicative of localization-related

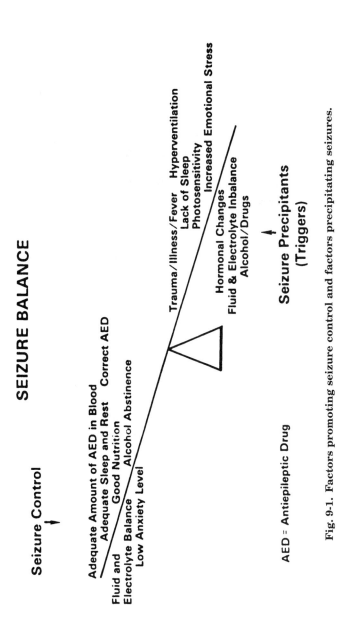

Fig. 9-1. Factors promoting seizure control and factors precipitating seizures.

epilepsy. Such findings include: facial asymmetry, asymmetry of thumb size (indicates contralateral cerebral damage during infancy or childhood), drift or pronation of outstretched hands, dystonic posture when walking on sides of feet, or naming difficulty (left temporal dysfunction). Finally, 3 minutes of good hyperventilation will usually produce absence seizures in untreated absence seizure patients.

VI. ELECTROENCEPHALOGRAM (EEG)

The EEG is a helpful diagnostic tool in the investigation of a seizure disorder. It confirms the presence of abnormal electrical activity, gives information regarding the type of seizure disorder, and discloses the location of the seizure focus. There are instances in which the routine EEG is normal, in spite of the fact that the patient has seizures or is suspected of having them. Under these circumstances, the study is repeated after the patient is deprived of sleep (4 hours or less of sleep the night before the study), and special (e.g., temporal or sphenoidal) leads may also be employed. This procedure is helpful in bringing out the abnormality in many cases, especially if discharges arise from the temporal lobe.

If the history unequivocally points to a seizure disorder, the patient should be treated despite a normal waking and sleep-deprived EEG. The usual EEG study samples only roughly an hour of time, and is normal in a significant percentage of patients with epilepsy. In cases in which it is not certain that a patient has seizures or the seizure type cannot be determined despite a careful history, physical examination, and routine waking and sleep-deprived EEG, the diagnosis often can be established by prolonged monitoring of the EEG.

VII. LABORATORY EXAMINATION (INCLUDING NEUROIMAGING)

Usually, the following laboratory tests should be performed in evaluating the cause of a newly diagnosed seizure disorder: metabolic screen, EEG recording in waking and sleep states, and magnetic resonance imaging (MRI, preferred) or computed tomographic (CT, acceptable) scan (see following). A toxic screen should be performed if alcohol or drug abuse or withdrawal is suspected. A lumbar puncture (for opening pressure, cell counts, protein, glucose, cytology, culture, and serology) should be performed if infection or malignancy is suspected.

The American Academy of Neurology has published (1996) practice parameters for neuroimaging (NI) studies (MRI, CT) of patients having a first seizure. Emergent NI (scan immediately) should be performed when a provider suspects a serious structural lesion. Clinical studies have shown a higher frequency of life-threatening lesions in patients with new focal deficits, persistent altered mental status (with or without intoxication), fever, recent trauma, persistent headache, history of cancer, history of anticoagulation, or suspicion of acquired immunodeficiency syndrome (AIDS).

Urgent NI (scan appointment is included in the disposition or is performed before disposition when follow-up of the patient's neurologic problem cannot be ensured) should be considered for patients who have completely recovered from their seizure and for whom no clear-cut cause has been identified (e.g., hypoglycemia, hyponatremia, tricyclic overdose) to help identify a possible structural cause. Because adequate follow-up is needed to ensure a patient's neurologic health, urgent NI may be obtained before disposition when timely follow-up cannot be ensured.

Additionally, for patients with first-time seizure, emergent NI should be considered if the patient is over 40 years of age or had partial onlet seizures.

Functional neuroimaging with position emission tomography and MRI are beyond the scope of this book. These topics have been reviewed in detail by George et al. (13) and Henry (15).

VIII. SYNTHESIS OF DATA

By combining history, physical examination, and EEG information it should be possible to determine: (a) the patient's events are seizures and (b) the patient's seizure type(s) according to the International Classification of Epileptic Seizures (Table 2-1). If this cannot be done, additional history (e.g., additional witnesses) and/or EEG (e.g., long-term EEG monitoring) information should be obtained. If all possible information has been gathered and the diagnosis remains uncertain, one usually is forced to act, based upon available history. If the history strongly suggests a recurrent seizure type, a therapeutic trial of antiepileptic medication appropriate for the

TABLE 9-1. Differential diagnosis of epilepsy at various ages

A.   All ages
  1. Epilepsy vs. migraine
  2. Epilepsy vs. syncope
  3. Epilepsy vs. Meniere's disease
  4. Epilepsy vs. episodic dyscontrol (rage attacks)
  5. Epilepsy vs. psychogenic seizure
  6. Absence seizures vs. complex partial seizures
B.   In children
  1. Epilepsy vs. movement disorder (tic, chorea, tremor)
  2. Epilepsy vs. cyanotic breath-holding spell
  3. Epilepsy vs. pallid infantile syncope
  4. Epilepsy vs. prolonged Q-T syndrome
  5. Epilepsy vs. sleep disturbance (night terrors, sleep walking)
  6. Epilepsy vs. abdominal migraine vs. intra-abdominal disease
C.   In adults
  1. Epilepsy vs. transient ischemic attack
  2. Epilepsy vs. Transient global amnesia

seizure type is usually begun. If the history does not strongly suggest recurrent seizures, observation without medication is the usual plan. Management of a patient having a single seizure is discussed in Chapter 10.

Seizure type combined with additional information from history, physical examination, EEG, and laboratory tests often allows one to determine the patient's specific epilepsy syndrome according to the International Classification of Epilepsies (Table 1-2 and Chapters 3–8). This determination assists with selection of therapy and counseling regarding prognosis and familial occurrence.

IX. DIFFERENTIAL DIAGNOSIS OF EPILEPSY

The common differential diagnostic problems with epilepsy at various ages are shown in Table 9-1, which also serves as an outline of this section. In each case, the two possible diagnoses have certain common features and certain unique features.

A. All Ages

1. Epilepsy vs. Migraine
   A. COMMON FEATURES. Episodic occurrence, headache, sensory (visual, paresthesias) or motor (weakness) aura, loss of consciousness (basilar migraine), and focal slowing on EEG are all common features of both epilepsy and migraine.

Both diseases are common and can occur in the same patient.

B. FEATURES SUGGESTING EPILEPSY. Headache absent or less severe, bilateral, and nonpulsatile; paroxysmal activity on interictal and ictal EEG (spikes, sharp waves, spike-waves); and persistent slowing on interictal EEG are features suggesting epilepsy.

C. FEATURES SUGGESTING MIGRAINE. Severe unilateral, pulsatile headache; nausea and vomiting; photophobia; family history of migraine; and EEG slowing only during or immediately after attack are features suggesting migraine.

D. OTHER. The neurologic auras of migraine may occur with or without headache. There is a large and conflicting literature on the EEG in migraine. Patients with only migraine may have paroxysmally abnormal EEGs. Abdominal epilepsy and abdominal migraine are discussed later in this chapter.

2. Epilepsy vs. Syncope

A. DEFINITIONS. *Syncope*, or fainting, is the sudden loss of muscle tone, collapse of posture, and loss of consciousness associated with a drop in systemic blood pressure. Syncopal attacks begin with a clouding of consciousness accompanied by vertigo, nausea, and a waxy pallor of the skin. The attack usually lasts approximately 10 sec.

Convulsive syncope has an onset similar to that of a typical syncopal attack. However, the onset is followed by a tonic spasm in which the back, head, and lower limbs are bent backward and the fists are clenched. This is often accompanied by mydriasis, nystagmus, drooling of saliva, and incontinence. The patient may bite his tongue, although this is rare.

The patient who falls to the floor quickly recovers from a faint when the blood pressure is re-established. If the person is unable to reach the supine position, as when fainting occurs in a chair or in a phone booth, cerebral circulation is re-established more slowly. Under these conditions convulsive syncope is more likely to occur.

B. DIFFERENTIAL DIAGNOSIS. See Table 9-2.

C. OTHER. Loss of postural tone, along with loss of consciousness, may cause falls which mimic syncope in absence, atonic, and complex partial seizures. Prolonged EEG and/or ECG monitoring is indicated when a differential diagnosis cannot be made on the basis of

TABLE 9-2. Differential diagnosis of seizure vs syncope

Clinical feature	Syncope	Seizure
Age of onset	Adult or child	Adult or child
Posture	Depends on initial condition or posture (erect)	Any posture
Muscle tone	Flaccid	Increased in tonic-clonic and some absence and complex partial seizures
Duration	10 sec	1–2 min (tonic-clonic); 1–3 min (complex partial); <15 sec (absence)
Sleep	Rarely occurs in sleep (but may if cardiac in origin)	May occur during sleep, upon awakening, or after sleep deprivation
Incontinence	Rarely	Often
Tongue biting or injury	Not likely with hypotonia	May occur during tonic phase
Skin color	Pale	Flushed
Respirations	Slow unless syncope is caused by hyperventilation	Apnea; stertorous
Perspiration	Cold, clammy	Hot, sweaty
EEG during event	Nonspecific slow	Specific paroxysms
EGG between events	Normal	Paroxysmal activity
ECG	May show arrhythmia, PVC, asystole, or other abnormality	Usually normal
Family history	Positive for syncope (sometimes)	Positive for seizure (sometimes)

criteria in Table 9-2. Note that one channel of a prolonged EEG recording can be devoted to ECG monitoring.

3. Epilepsy vs. Meniere's Disease

A. COMMON FEATURES. Episodic vertigo and/or tinnitus can occur on both. Interictal EEG abnormal in 25% of Meniere's disease patients (temporal slowing).

B. FEATURES SUGGESTING EPILEPSY. Other symptoms of simple partial or complex seizures of lateral temporal origin (altered consciousness, language disorders, visual misperceptions); and sharp waves or spikes on interictal EEG.

C. FEATURES SUGGESTING MENIERE'S DISEASE. Hearing loss.

4. Epilepsy vs. Episodic Dyscontrol (Rage Attacks)

A. DEFINITIONS. The episodic dyscontrol syndrome is characterized by recurrent attacks of uncontrollable rage and/or aggression (verbal or physical). Of particular note, attacks typically have an identifiable precipitant, although the severity of the precipitant typically does not justify the severity of the attack. The syndrome is usually seen in teenagers and young adults, but can be seen in younger children and older adults. Many patients have an irritable personality between attacks. In many patients, neurologic impairment is evident on neurologic examination. In particular, there may be evidence of ventromedial frontal lobe impairment because this area is involved in measuring behavioral response to environmental stimuli. The diagnosis is based on the history provided by patients, relatives, and onlookers. The patient's attacks occur suddenly and can be explosive and characterized by uncontrollable behavior, consisting of verbal aggression and/or physical violence such as kicking, gouging, scratching, spitting, hitting, and biting. In girls and women, the violence is frequently verbal and consists of obscene, profane language. Patients often display remarkable strength and speed in their attacks. During the attacks the patients often appear temporarily psychotic and after the attacks amnesia, fatigue, and, occasionally, remorse may occur. Finally, it is not uncommon for episodic dyscontrol syndrome and real partial seizures to exist in the same patient because they both are consequences of brain damage (especially in head injury patients).

B. DIFFERENTIAL DIAGNOSIS. See Table 9-3.

5. Epilepsy vs. Psychogenic Seizures

A. EXTENT OF PROBLEM. Psychogenic seizures are more common than generally realized. Ten to thirty percent of persons referred to epilepsy centers for "medically refractory" epilepsy have psychogenic seizures. Approximately one-half of patients with psychogenic seizures also have "real" seizures, making management particularly complex.

B. DEFINITION. Psychogenic seizures are episodes of altered movement, emotion, sensation, or experience which are similar to those caused by epilepsy, but which have purely emotional causes. Psychogenic seizures may mimic any seizure type, but tonic-clonic and complex partial are the most common types mimicked. Psychogenic seizures may be deliberate, willed acts (malingering) to gain a desired end. Prisoners and persons receiving compensation for seizures sometimes

TABLE 9-3. Epilepsy vs episodic dyscontrol (rage attacks)

Clinical data	Episodic dyscontrol	Epilepsy[a]
Precipitating factors	Almost always	Occasionally
Warning	No	May have aura
Violence	Frequently, often person-directed	Rarely, almost never person-directed
Stereotype of attacks	Variable	Usually stereotyped
Incontinence	Rarely	Occasionally
Self-injury	Occasionally	Occasionally
Amnesia for event	Often	Usually for part of attack
Postictal symptoms	Frequently exhausted, confused	Usually tired, disoriented, confused
Interictal behavioral abnormalities	Frequently	Occasionally
Response to AEDs	Variable	Variable
EEG		
Interictal	Frequently abnormal	Frequently abnormal
Ictal	No change	Epileptiform discharges

[a]Complex partial seizures.

fall into this category. Psychogenic seizures may also be subconscious acts. Persons with limited intelligence and/or persons with a history of physical or sexual abuse may use psychogenic seizures as a "cry for help." Persons with normal intelligence may use psychogenic seizures to control their environment.

C. **DIFFERENTIAL DIAGNOSIS.** See Table 9-4.

D. **OTHER.** In patients having both psychogenic and "real" seizures, the psychogenic seizures have the features of psychogenic seizures listed in Table 9-4. The "real" seizures have the features of "real" seizures listed in Table 9-4. See Devinsky, et al. (10) for further discussion of this difficult group of patients. The best differential diagnostic test is to record a typical attack with EEG and video monitoring. Clinical features can be carefully observed. The EEG is abnormal during all tonic-clonic seizures, 90% of complex partial seizures, and only 50% of simple partial seizures.

Serum prolactin levels are reliably (91%) elevated after tonic-clonic seizures, but not after psychogenic or complex partial seizures. A sample must be obtained within 10 min of the seizure and again in 90 to 120 min (control). An elevation of 2.5 times over control suggests a tonic-clonic seizure.

Lesser (16) has recently performed a complete review of psychogenic seizures.

6. Absence Seizures vs. Complex Partial Seizures

A. COMMON FEATURES. Intermittent loss of consciousness, sometimes with automatisms. Both seizure types occur in children and adults.

B. DIFFERENTIAL DIAGNOSIS. See Table 9-5.

C. OTHER. There is a mistaken tendency for diagnosing physicians to call lapses of consciousness in children absence seizures, and lapses in consciousness in adults complex partial seizures. Both seizure types occur in both age groups.

B. In Children

1. Epilepsy vs. Movement Disorder (Tic, Chorea, Tremor)

On occasion, movement disorders such as *tics and chorea* may be confused with partial motor seizures. In children, tics involve primarily the head, neck, and shoulders and consist of complex movements such as facial grimacing, eye blinking or rolling, head nodding or turning, and shrugging of the shoulders. Tics can usually be suppressed, at least temporarily, by an effort of will, whereas seizures cannot. In chorea, the movements occur randomly, usually in multiple muscle groups, whereas seizures are usually characterized by repetitive, stereotyped movements affecting the same muscle groups. Seizures do not have the characteristic, continuous flow of movements that is so distinctive of chorea. *Tremors* can usually be differentiated from seizures by the smooth to-and-fro movements compared with seizures, which are more abrupt and have distinct intervals between each movement.

2. Epilepsy vs. Cyanotic Breath-Holding Spells

A. DEFINITIONS. Such spells typically begin with some type of distressing event to the child, either frustration, fright, or minor injuries, such as mild blows, cuts, bumps, or spankings. The elements of unexpectedness and surprise are often present. The child then begins to vigorously cry. After the first few cries, the child suddenly gasps, holds his breath, and becomes cyanotic, most prominently around the lips. The child then becomes rigid, loses consciousness, and may assume an opisthotonic posture. Shortly thereafter, the child loses muscle tone and remains limp until normal breathing is

TABLE 9-4. Epilepsy vs. psychogenic seizures

Epilepsy	Psychogenic seizures
Neutral setting	Emotionally charged setting
Stereotyped, with minor variations among attacks	Sometimes rigidly stereotyped; sometimes variable and affected by environment
Abrupt onset and end of attack	Gradual build-up and prolonged resolution
Tongue biting, incontinence, postictal confusion often present	Tongue biting, incontinence, postictal confusion may be present
Self-injury common	Self-injury rare
Family history of typical epileptic phenomena	May have epilepsy in family
Fragmentary recall or no recall of event	Indifference, apparent amnesia for event
Desire to know about attack, to replace lost time (ego-alien)	Denial of details and unwillingness to consider motivational determinants
Secondary gain usually lacking	Secondary gains often identifiable
Abnormal interictal EEG (most)	Normal interictal EEG (63–73%)
General features	
Specific precipitant: Rare	Specific precipitant: Common (often stress)
Onset: Usually short	Onset: Often gradual
Inability to respond or abort attack	Ability to respond or abort attack
Eyes open	Eyes forcefully closed
Injury: Common	Injury: Less common
Urination: May occur	Urination: May occur
Defecation: May occur	Defecation: May occur

TABLE 9-4. *Continued*

Epilepsy	*Psychogenic seizures*
Tonic-clonic seizure	
Mouth open during tonic phase	Mouth closed during tonic phase
Onset with vocalization and tonic phase	Side-to-side neck movements
Followed by synchronous clonic movements	Nonsynchronous movements
Followed by flaccid coma	Pelvic thrusting
Duration of 2 min or less	Prolonged motor activity
	No rigidity
	Vocalization throughout attack
	Variable duration
Complex partial seizure	
Onset with epigastric sensation: special senses sensation; behavioral changes: unilateral sensory or motor symptoms	Onset with behavioral changes, hyperventilation, headache, dizziness
Onset with motionless stare	Variable duration
Vocalization: simple, often repetitive	Vocalization: complex
Duration 1–3 min	Directed violence

TABLE 9-5. Differential diagnosis of absence vs. complex partial seizures

	Absence	*Complex partial*
Age of onset	Childhood	Any age, relatively rare in childhood
Aura	None	Common
Seizure		
Duration	Seconds	Minutes
Alertness	Out of contact	Out of contact
Automatisms	Simple or complex	Simple or complex
Staring	Yes	Yes
Speech	Never formed; patient sometimes hums	Incoherent, dysphasic, or none
Postictal confusion	Never	Often
Amnesia for attack	Yes	Yes, some islands of memory
Precipitation by hyperventilation	Often	Rarely
Precipitation by photic stimulation	Sometimes	Very rarely
EEG	3-Hz spike-wave	Temporal slowing or sharp activity

restored. The child regains composure rapidly, and the marked lethargy and confusion seen after a generalized tonic or tonic-clonic seizure usually do not occur. Usually the period of breath-holding is brief and may be associated with a very brief period of cyanosis. However, if the apnea results in significant hypoxia, a brief generalized tonic-clonic seizure may ensue. Even when the child has a convulsion as a component of the breath-holding attack, the postictal phase is very brief. Most breath-holding episodes last a minute or less.

The majority of children begin having breath-holding spells between the ages of 6 and 18 months. It is not rare, however, for breath-holding spells to have their onset in the first weeks of life. Approximately 5% of children have the onset of breath-holding attacks after 2 years of age. The children usually have normal neurologic and developmental examinations.

B. DIFFERENTIAL DIAGNOSIS. See Table 9-6.

3. Epilepsy vs. Pallid Infantile Syncope

A. DEFINITIONS. These events, also termed reflex anoxic seizures, vagal attacks, or white breath-holding, are less common than cyanotic breath-holding attacks. Like cyanotic breath-holding attacks, pallid infantile syncope

TABLE 9-6. Differentiation of breath-holding atttacks and pallid infantile syncope from generalized tonic or tonic-clonic seizures

Clinical data	Cyanotic breath-holding	Pallid infantile syncope	Seizures: tonic-clonic or tonic
Age	6 mos–6 yrs	12–18 mos; highly variable	Any age
Precipitating factors	Almost always	Almost always	Occasionally
Family history	Frequently positive for breath-holding	Frequently positive for syncope	Frequently positive for seizures
Sequence of events	Crying—apnea—loss of consciousness	Upset—pallor—loss of consciousness	Aura—loss of consciousness
Heart rate during ocular compression	Bradycardia or no change	Marked bradycardia or asystole	Physiologic tachycardia
Postictal symptoms	Usually none	Usually none	Always with GTC, usually brief symptoms with tonic
EEG:			
Interictal	Normal	Normal	Usually abnormal
Ictal	Slowing	Slowing	Epileptiform activity

is precipitated by a stressful situation such as unexpected pain. A few seconds after the provocation the child suddenly falls limply to the ground. Crying before the loss of consciousness may or may not be present. The child then either quickly regains consciousness or, in more severe cases, convulsions may occur. While cyanosis may occur, it is not as prominent as during cyanotic breath-holding spells. Pallor and cold sweats may precede the loss of consciousness. Although not always obvious to the observer, the child usually does not breathe during the initial phase of the attack. As with cyanotic breath-holding attacks, children usually recover quickly from pallid infantile syncope.

The age range for pallid infantile syncope is broader than cyanotic breath-holding spells, varying from 3 months to 14 years, with a median age of 4 years. The disorder is especially common between the ages of 12 and 18 months when the onset of walking is associated with frequent falls.

At one time, *ocular compression* was commonly performed to aide in the diagnosis of pallid infantile syncope and breath-holding attacks. During EKG and EEG monitoring, pressure on the ocular globe was applied. Asystole, of 2 seconds' or greater duration, occurred in over one-half of children with pallid infantile syncope and one-fourth of those with cyanotic breath-holding. In cases in which asystole lasted 10 seconds or more, a typical anoxic seizure followed a period of unconsciousness with decerebrate posturing and extension of all limbs. While some laboratories continue to use this procedure, most clinicians rely on the history for the diagnosis. Table 9-6 lists the differentiating features of cyanotic breath-holding, pallid infantile syncope, and generalized tonic-clonic seizures.

B. DIFFERENTIAL DIAGNOSIS. See Table 9-6.

4. Epilepsy vs. Prolonged Q-T Syndrome

This syndrome can mimic idiopathic epilepsy. This is a serious disorder that can lead to ventricular fibrillation or tachycardia. Any child with unexplained episodes of loss of consciousness should have an EKG. This is especially important if there is a positive family history or if the loss of consciousness was induced by exercise, fright, or excitement.

5. Epilepsy vs. Sleep Disturbance (Night Terror, Sleep Walking)

A. COMMON FEATURES (WITH COMPLEX PARTIAL SEIZURES). Recurrence in sleep, prominent fear and autonomic phenomena (night terrors), automatic behavior, and amnesia for event.

B. FEATURES SUGGESTING NIGHT TERRORS. Onset between 4 and 12 years of age, typical spell begins 1 to 2 hr after falling asleep (stages 3 and 4 sleep), terrified scream, child appears panic-stricken and confused, tachypnea, diaphoresis, dilated pupils often present, fearful for up to 15 min then falls back to sleep without difficulty, normal EEG.

C. FEATURES SUGGESTING SLEEP WALKING. Typical spell begins 1 to 2 hr after falling asleep (stages 3 and 4 sleep); walks about in a trance and may carry out purposeful activity such as dressing, opening doors, and eating; *somnilogny* or *sleep talking* may occur independently or with sleep walking; normal EEG.

D. FEATURES SUGGESTING COMPLEX PARTIAL SEIZURES. Occurrence shortly after going to bed at night or in the early morning hours (stages 1 or 2 sleep); other clinical features of complex partial seizures; sharp waves or spikes on interictal EEG.

6. Abdominal Epilepsy vs. Abdominal Migraine vs. Intra-abdominal Disease

A. COMMON FEATURES. Recurrent abdominal pain with vomiting and other autonomic signs and symptoms; childhood occurrence.

B. FEATURES SUGGESTING EPILEPSY. Other clinical features of simple or complex partial seizures (may not be present); sharp waves or spikes on interictal EEG; response to antiepileptic drugs.

C. FEATURES SUGGESTING MIGRAINE. Other clinical features of migraine (may not be present); family history of migraine; response to antimigraine drugs.

D. OTHER. Most children with recurrent abdominal pain do not have epilepsy or migraine. Other causes should be sought vigorously.

C. In Adults

1. Epilepsy vs. Transient Ischemic Attack (TIA)

A. COMMON FEATURES. Both partial seizures and TIAs often begin at older age. Transient sensory, motor, speech, vestibular, or memory symptoms may occur with either. Both typically last only a few minutes.

B. FEATURES SUGGESTING EPILEPSY. Younger age (but not uncommon in elderly).Other signs or symptoms of partial seizures (motor, sensory, autonomic, or psychic);

alteration of consciousness; automatisms; postictal confusion; hemianopic, scotomatous, or positive (lights, colors) visual symptoms; duration less than 3 min; focal spikes or slowing on interictal EEG.

C. FEATURES SUGGESTING TIA. Duration longer than 3 min (may be briefer); monocular blindness; signs or symptoms suggesting carotid artery distribution deficit (hemiparesis, hemisensory loss, neglect of one side, aphasia); signs or symptoms suggesting vertebral artery distribution deficit (vertigo, diplopia, dysphagia, dysarthria, deafness, drop attacks); cardiovascular risk factors (may be present in older patient with seizures); carotid bruit, decreased pulse (may be present in older patient with seizures); normal interictal EEG.

2. Transient Global Amnesia

Transient global amnesia usually occurs in patients over 50 years of age. There is sudden onset of amnesia lasting for several hours. Patients are alert with fluent speech but are confused. Recurrent attacks may occur in up to 25% of patients. There is an ongoing debate as to whether these attacks are of vascular origin and/or seizure origin. They usually are not treated with antiepileptic drugs unless paroxysmal activity is found on the EEG.

REFERENCES

1. American Academy of Neurology Quality Standards Subcommittee. Practice parameter: neuroimaging in the emergency patient presenting with seizure-summary statement. *Neurology* 1996;47:280–291.
2. Anderman F. Overview: disorders that can be confused with epilepsy. In: Engel J, Pedley TA, eds. *Epilepsy: a comprehensive textbook.* Philadelphia: Lippincott–Raven, 1997.
3. Barnett HJM, Mohr JP, Stein BM, et al., (eds). *Stroke: pathophysiology, diagnosis and management*, 2nd ed. New York: Churchill Livingston, 1992.
4. Breningstall G. Breath holding spells. *Pediatric Neurology* 1996;14:91–97.
5. Browne TR, Feldman RG. Epilepsy an overview. In: Browne TR, Feldman RG, eds. *Epilepsy: diagnosis and management.* Boston: Little Brown, 1983.
6. Carpay JA, deWeed AW, Schimsheiner RJ, et al. The diagnostic yield of a second EEG after partial sleep deprivation: a prospective study in children with newly diagnosed seizures. *Epilepsia* 1997;38:595–599.

7. Commission on Classification and Terminology of the International League Against Epilepsy. Proposal for revised clinical and electrocephalographic classification of epileptic seizures. *Epilepsia* 1981;22:489–501.

8. Commission on Classification and Terminology of the International League Against Epilepsy. Proposal for revised classification of epilepsies and epileptic syndromes. *Epilepsia* 1989;30:389–399.

9. Daly DD. The EEG in epilepsy and syncope. In: Daly DD, Pedley TA, eds. *Current practice of clinical electroencephalography,* 2nd ed. New York: Raven Press, 1990.

10. Devinsky O, Sauchez-Villasenor F, Vasquez B, et al. Clinical profile of patients with epileptic and nonepileptic seizures. *Neurology* 1996;46:1530–1533.

11. Engel J, Pedley TA, eds. *Epilepsy: a comprehensive textbook.* Philadelphia: Lippincott–Raven, 1997, Chapters 70–93, 253–270.

12. Grafman J, Schwab K, Waren D, et al. Frontal lobe injuries, violence, and aggression. *Neurology* 1996;46:1231–1238.

13. George, JS, Aine CJ, Mosner JC, et al. Mapping function in the human brain with magnetoencephalography, anatomical magnetic resonance imaging, and functional magnetic resonance imaging. *J Clin Neurophysiol* 1996;12;406–431.

14. Hauser WA, Hesdorffer DC. *Epilepsy: frequency, causes and consequences.* New York: Demos, 1990.

15. Henry TR. Progress in epilepsy research: functional neuroimaging with position emission tomography. *Epilepsia* 1996;37:1141–1154.

16. Lesser RP. Psychogenic seizures. *Neurology* 1996;46:1499–1507.

17. Miller JW, Petersen RC, Metter EJ, et al. Transient global amnesia. *Neurology* 1987;37:733–737.

18. Moshe SL, Pedley TA. Overview: diagnostic evaluation. In: Engel J, Pedley TA, eds. *Epilepsy: a comprehensive textbook.* Philadelphia: Lippincott–Raven, 1997.

19. Son K, Anderman F. Differential diagnosis. In: Engel J, Pedley TA, eds. *Epilepsy: a comprehensive textbook.* Philadelphia: Lippincott–Raven, 1997.

20. Wyllie E, ed. *The treatment of epilepsy: principles and practice,* 2nd ed. Baltimore: Williams and Wilkins, 1997, Chapters 14–20, 47, 48.

21. Wyllie E, ed. Neuroimaging and epilepsy: the role of new techniques. *Epilepsia* 1994;(suppl 6):35.

MANAGEMENT

I. ESTABLISH DIAGNOSIS

The first step in managing epilepsy is to correctly determine seizure type, epileptic syndrome, etiology and precipitating factors. This process is described in Chapter 9.

II. IDENTIFY AND DEAL WITH PSYCHOLOGICAL AND SOCIAL PROBLEMS

Seizures are a relatively rare phenomenon for most patients. The psychological consequences of having epilepsy, however, are present all the time. Loss of one's driver's license, employment, self-esteem, and position in peer groups are all potential problems and may cause more suffering than the seizures themselves. Furthermore, the anxiety associated with these psychological problems of epilepsy may precipitate seizures in some patients. One must anticipate that the patient will experience psychological problems as a consequence of having epilepsy. Also, one must be prepared to assist the patient by carefully explaining the nature of the medical problems and the effect the problems will have on driving and employment by providing emotional support, by giving the patient an opportunity to talk through his or her problems, and by referring the patient to various resources available to assist the patient with epilepsy (e.g., social workers, epilepsy societies, vocational counselors). For more details see Chapter 14 or Moshe et al. (16).

III. PRINCIPLES OF PHARMACOLOGIC THERAPY

A. Begin Monotherapy with Drug of Choice

Once the exact type of seizure has been determined, the physician should initiate monotherapy (single-drug therapy) with the drug that has shown the best combination of high efficacy and low toxicity in comparative studies of drugs for the patient's seizure type (Table 10-1). If a patient has more than one type of seizure, therapy should begin with the drug of choice for the combination of seizure types present (Table 10-1). Reasons for selection of specific drugs as drugs of choice for specific seizure types are given in Section IV.

The single-drug approach for initial treatment is preferred because monotherapy with an appropriately selec-

TABLE 10-1. Antiepileptic drugs of choice

Seizure type	Drug(s) of first choice[a]	Drug(s) of second choice[a]	Alternative drug(s)[a]
Partial (simple, complex, secondarily generalized tonic-clonic)	Carbamazepine Phenytoin	Gabapentin Lamotrigine, Topiramate Valproic acid	Phenobarbital Primidone
Primarily generalized tonic-clonic	Phenytoin Valproic acid[b]	Carbamazepine	Phenobarbital Primidone
Absence	Ethosuximide Valproic acid[b]	Valproic acid	Clonazepam Lamotrigine

[a]Listed alphabetically within groups.
[b]Used if combination of absence and tonic-clonic seizures present.

ted drug pushed to the adequate dosing rate will control seizures in 70% to 90% of patients, and polytherapy (more than one drug therapy) exposes the patient to several unnecessary risks. Factors that appear to be associated with failure of monotherapy include: persistent noncompliance, drug allergy, large or progressive brain lesions, partial seizures, more than one type of seizure, neuropsychiatric handicaps, and high pretreatment seizure frequency.

The risks of unnecessary polytherapy are many. Chronic toxicity is associated with the use of any antiepileptic drug. Polytherapy may include barbiturates, which are associated with high risk for cognitive and behavioral toxicity. Other risks of unnecessary polytherapy include drug allergy, drug interactions, exacerbation of seizures, and the inability to evaluate the effectiveness of individual antiepileptic drugs.

B. Push the First Drug Tried

The first drug tried for a seizure disorder is usually among the least toxic drugs available, and the physician must be certain that he or she has obtained the maximum possible therapeutic effect from the first drug before adding other drugs. Therapy usually begins with a so-called "average" dosage of antiepileptic drug. If the seizures are controlled with this average dosage and there are no serious side effects, no further changes are necessary. If the seizures are not controlled with this dosage, and there is no serious drug toxicity, the dosage of the drug should be systematically increased until the seizures are controlled or until side effects preclude further dosage increase.

The drug-plasma concentration should be determined if a patient's seizures are not controlled by an average or high drug dosage. There are many correctable causes of lower than expected drug-plasma concentration, including inadequate dosing rate, noncompliance, poor absorption, drug interactions, generic drug substitutions, pregnancy, and patient error. It would be a serious error to substitute or to add a more toxic drug because the patient has a low plasma concentration of the first drug. A drug cannot be said to be ineffective until it is documented that the seizures are not controlled with a high therapeutic plasma concentration of the drug, unless drug toxicity precludes reaching such concentrations.

The therapeutic range of drug-plasma concentration represents values applicable to average patients. Some patients require higher drug-plasma concentrations than the therapeutic range for good seizure control. If a patient has a high therapeutic plasma concentration of a nontoxic drug, poor seizure control, and no drug side effects, the best approach usually is to increase the dosage of the first drug rather than add a more toxic second drug.

C. Add Additional Drugs

If the first drug is pushed to its maximum tolerated dosage and seizures still are not controlled, a second antiepileptic drug should be added. In general, it is best to add the second drug and continue administration of the first drug (at least temporarily) because (a) the first drug will provide protection while the plasma concentration of the second drug is being built up; (b) discontinuing the first drug may result in withdrawal activation of the seizure disorder; and (c) there is evidence that two antiepileptic drugs in combination may control seizures in some patients when either drug alone does not.

When a therapeutic plasma concentration of the second drug is obtained, the physician should consider tapering the patient off the first drug because of the many hazards of chronic polytherapy. The decision to taper the patient off the first drug must be individualized and should take into consideration the antiepileptic effect of the first drug when it is given alone, the side effects of the first drug, and the psychosocial consequences to the patient of having a seizure if withdrawal of the first drug results in loss of complete seizure control. The adverse effects of antiepileptic drugs on behavior and cognition argue that one should attempt to minimize the number of these drugs given to children. In adults, the hazards of polytherapy must be weighed against the risk of loss of job, driver's license, or both if withdrawal of the first drug results in a recurrence of seizures. If it is elected to withdraw the first drug, the withdrawal should be done slowly (discussed in detail further on).

A third drug should not be added until it is documented that seizures cannot be controlled with maximum tolerated doses of the first two drugs tried. It is usually better to add a third drug (at least temporarily) than to substitute the third drug for the first or second drug, for reasons similar to those cited earlier for adding, rather than substituting, the second drug. After a therapeutic plasma concentration of the third drug is reached, the physician may elect to withdraw one of the first two drugs, using the guidelines outlined earlier.

IV. DRUGS OF CHOICE

A. First Choice Drugs for Simple Partial, Complex, Partial and Secondarily Generalized Tonic-Clonic Seizures

Simple partial (focal), complex partial (psychomotor, temporal lobe), and tonic-clonic (grand mal) seizures are the most common types of seizure disorders and occur at all ages. Note that a tonic-clonic seizure may be focal (partial seizures secondarily generalized) or generalized (primarily generalized) in onset (see Chapter 2). Carbamazepine (Tegretol), phenobarbital, phenytoin (Dilantin), primidone (Mysoline), and valproic acid (Depakote) are the drugs that have been employed as initial therapy for simple partial, complex partial, and partial seizures secondarily generalized. These five drugs have been compared in adults in two large Veterans Administration Cooperative studies. Primidone was inferior to the other four drugs for all seizure types because of a significantly higher incidence of intolerable toxicity.

Carbamazepine and phenytoin are the two drugs of choice for partial seizures and partial seizures secondarily generalized in adults based on the following data: (a) carbamazepine and phenytoin have fewer side effects than phenobarbital or valproic acid, regardless of seizure type; (b) carbamazepine and phenytoin are more effective than phenobarbital or valproic acid for complex partial seizures; (c) there were no statistically significant differences in efficacy or toxicity when carbamazepine was compared with phenytoin; and (d) monotherapy with carbamazepine or phenytoin will produce a satisfactory long-term result in approximately 80% of patients.

In children, comparative studies have demonstrated that carbamazepine, phenytoin, and valproic acid are equally efficacious. Phenobarbital and primidone also are efficacious, but side effects such as irritability, hyperactivity, and lethargy limit these drugs to second-line therapy.

Four new drugs have been approved by the FDA since 1993 for partial seizures: felbamate (Felbatol), gabapentin (Neurontin), lamotrigine (Lamictal), and topiramate (Topamax). Only felbamate is FDA-approved as initial therapy for these seizure types; but felbamate never is used now as initial therapy because of the risks of aplastic anemia and liver failure. All four new drugs are approved for use when first-choice drugs fail (see following). There are published studies indicating gabapentin and lamotrigine may have efficacy and safety similar to carbamazepine, when used as initial monotherapy.

B. Second Choice Drugs for Simple Partial, Complex Partial and Secondarily Generalized Tonic-Clonic Seizures

There are no definitive published trials establishing the drug of second choice for patients failing a trial with a first-choice drug (carbamazepine or phenytoin). Probably the most common practice is to add or substitute (see earlier) the other first-choice drug based on results of initial therapy studies.

This practice has been questioned because: (a) carbamazepine and phenytoin have complex drug interactions when taken together; and (b) both drugs have the same mechanism of action.

Three older drugs (phenobarbital, primidone, valproic acid) and three new drugs (gabapentin, lamotrigine, topiramate) have been used as alternative drugs in patients failing to respond to carbamazepine, phenytoin, or both.

The advantages and disadvantages of these drugs are summarized in Table 10-2. Phenobarbital and primidone have fallen from favor because of high incidence of cognitive/behavioral side effects and drug interactions. Although used by many experts, valproic acid is not more effective than newer agents and has more problems with serious toxicity, nuisance toxicity, and drug interactions.

Gabapentin has no serious drug toxicity, little nuisance toxicity, and no drug interactions. Lamotrigine is

TABLE 10-2. Adjunctive medications for partial seizures

	Responder rate[a]	No serious toxicity	No nuisance toxicity	No drug interactions	Administration
Gabapentin	30–40%	+	±	+	t.i.d.
Lamotrigine	30–40%	–	±	±	b.i.d.
Phenobarbital	?[b]	+	–	–	q.d.
Primidone	?[b]	+	–	–	t.i.d.
Topiramate	40–50%	–	–	+	b.i.d.
Valproic acid	30–40%	–	–	–	b.i.d. or t.i.d.

[a]Percent of patients having a 50% or greater reduction in partial seizure frequency.
[b]Not determined in a modern, controlled study.

well-tolerated by many patients and has few drug interactions with non-antiepileptic drugs. Topiramate has the highest reported responder rate and few drug interactions.

C. Drugs for Primary Generalized Tonic-Clonic Seizures

For primarily generalized tonic-clonic seizures, carbamazepine, phenytoin, and valproic acid are all highly effective. Valproic acid has efficacy against absence and myoclonic seizures (sometimes associated with primarily generalized tonic-clonic seizures), whereas carbamazepine and phenytoin do not. Absence seizures may worsen in some patients taking carbamazepine or phenobarbital. Valproic acid is the drug of first choice for persons with primarily generalized tonic-clonic plus absence and/or myoclonic seizures.

D. Antiepileptic Drugs of Choice for Absence Seizures

Ethosuximide, valproic acid, and clonazepam are the three drugs used to treat absence seizures (see Table 10-1) and are equally effective for absence seizures. Ethosuximide has the fewest side effects and is the first-choice drug for uncomplicated absence seizures. For patients having tonic-clonic and/or myoclonic seizures in addition to absence seizures, valproic acid is the drug of first choice (ethosuximide has no efficacy for tonic-clonic or myoclonic seizures). Lamotrigine appears to be a promising new drug for absences.

V. SINGLE SEIZURE

Epilepsy by definition is recurring spontaneous seizures. Epilepsy must begin with a first seizure, but not all first seizures mean the beginning of epilepsy. Three-quarters of persons with an isolated seizure never have another.

A single first seizures may be caused by: (a) external events affecting a normal brain (e.g., drug toxicity, drug withdrawal, sleep deprivation); (b) somatic disease which transiently affects a normal brain (e.g., hypoglycemia, hypoxia, syncope, hyponatremia); (c) a neurologic disease injuring the brain (e.g., head injury, stroke, neoplasm); and (d) a first seizure as part of symptomatic or idiopathic epilepsy. Etiologies 1 and 2 are not indicative of recurring spontaneous seizures and do not require chronic antiepileptic drug treatment. Etiologies 3 and 4 are associated with risk of recurring spontaneous seizures.

Factors increasing risk for recurring seizures include: (a) evidence of structural lesion (strongest predictor); (b) abnormal electroencephalogram (EEG); (c) partial seizure type; (d) positive family history; and (e) postictal motor paralysis. Persons with no risk factors have only a 15% chance of a second seizure within 2 years. Persons with two or more risk factors have a 100% chance of seizure recurrence within 2 years.

Antiepileptic drug therapy with therapeutic blood levels has been shown to reduce the risk of seizure recurrence after a first seizure. Persons with two or more risk factors probably should be treated. Other patients may not be obligated to be treated, but should be warned of the risk of recurrent seizures (especially in the next 2 years) and appropriate precautions advised.

VI. DRUG INTERACTIONS

Four forms of clinically important drug interactions have been found with antiepileptic drugs: (a) induction of biotransformation of coadministered drug; (b) inhibition of biotransformation of coadministered drug; (c) displacement from protein-binding sites of coadministration of drug; and (d) pharmacodynamic interactions (both drugs affect common receptor sites, drug-plasma concentration unchanged). Drug interactions may be bidirectional (i.e., the both drugs are affected by the presence of the other drug), and one drug may have more than one type of drug interaction with the other drug. The mechanistic and clin-

TABLE 10-3. Common drug interactions of antiepileptic drugs

Carbamazapine (Tegretol)
Effect of adding carbamazepine to other drug

↑ Level of:	Phenytoin
↓ Level of:	Theophylline
	Valproic acid
	Oral contraceptives
	Lamotrigine

Effect of adding other drugs to carbamazepine

↑ Carbamazepine level:	Erythromycin
	Izoniazid
	Verapamil
↓ Carbamazepine level:	Phenytoin
	Phenobarbital
	Primidone

Gabapentin (Neurotin)
None unless drug alters glomerular filtration
None clinically significant

Lamotrigine (Lamictal)
Effect of adding lamotrigine to other drug
  ↑ Toxicity of carbamazepine
    (? pharmacodynamic)
Effect of adding other drug to lamotrigine
  ↑ Lamotrigine level: Valproic acid
Effect of adding other drug to lamotrigine

↓ Lamotrigine level:	Carbamazepine
	Phenobarbital
	Phenytoin

Phenobarbital
Effect of adding phenobarbital to other drug

↓ Level of:	Oral contraceptives
	Warfarin
	Theophylline
	Cimetadine
	Valproic acid
	Carbamazepine
	Lamotrigine

ical aspects of antiepileptic drug interactions have been reviewed in depth elsewhere [Levy and Bourgeois (13)].

Common drug interactions between antiepileptic drugs and between antiepileptic drugs and other types of drugs are listed in Table 10-3. Other less common drug interactions have been reported. Whenever an additional drug of any type is to be added to a patient's antiepileptic drug regimen, it is prudent to consult a listing of possible drug interactions such as that of Tatro (18).

TABLE 10-3. *Continued*

Effect of adding other drug to phenobarbital
  ↑ Phenobarbital level: Valproic acid

Phenytoin (Dilantin)
Effects of adding phenytoin to other drugs

↑ Level of:	Warfarin
↓ Level of:	Methadone
	Theophylline
	Carbamazepine
	Valproic acid
	Oral contraceptives
	Lamotrigine

Effects of adding other drug to phenytoin

↑ Phenytoin level:	Chloramphenicol
	Izoniazid
	Cimetadine
	Carbamazepine
	Disulfiram
↓ Phenytoin level:	AlOH, MgOH, $CaCO_3$ Antacids
	Valproic acid (free phenytoin unchanged)

Valproic acid (Depakote)
Effect of adding valproic acid to other drug

↑ Level of:	Phenobarbital
	Lamotrigine

Effect of adding other drug to valproic acid

↓ Valproic acid level:	Carbamazepine
	Phenobarbital
	Phenytoin

Topiramate (Topamax)
Effect of adding topiramate to other drug

↑ Level of:	Phenytoin
↓ Level of:	Valproic acid

Effect of adding other drug to topiramate

↓ Topiramate level:	Carbamazepine
	Phenytoin
	Valproic acid

VII. ANTIEPILEPTIC DRUG-PLASMA CONCENTRATION DETERMINATIONS ("BLOOD LEVELS")

A. Definitions

Plasma concentration of a drug refers to the amount of drug (by weight) dissolved in a unit volume of plasma. "Blood level" is a term often used as a synonym for plasma concentration.

B. Units

The units for antiepileptic drug-plasma concentration determinations most widely used in the United States are weight-per-volume units, such as micrograms per milliliter (µg/ml). In Europe and many other areas of the world molar units are used. The most widely used molar unit is micromoles (µmoles). A conversion table for weight-per-volume to molar units is given in the Appendix.

C. Indications for Determining Antiepileptic Drug-Plasma Concentration

1. Poor Seizure Control

Poor seizure control is the most frequent indication for obtaining antiepileptic drug-plasma concentration determinations. Use of such determinations may decrease by as much as 50% the number of patients whose seizures are poorly controlled when compared with patients whose therapy is empirically determined.

When a patient's seizures are not controlled with an average dosage of an antiepileptic drug appropriate for the type of seizure being treated, the plasma concentration of the drug should be determined. The first drug used in treating a given patient's seizure disorder is usually chosen because the drug should have the best efficacy-to-toxicity ratio for the patient. There are many causes for a lower than expected drug-plasma concentration, and these causes can often be identified and corrected (see following).

2. Initiation of Drug Therapy, Dosage Adjustment, Change in Concomitant Medication

In each of these situations, it may be wise to determine the plasma concentration of an antiepileptic drug to determine if it is within the desired range. One must allow sufficient time for steady-state plasma concentration to be attained after any change in drug regimen (see Table 11-1).

3. Evaluation of Antiepileptic Drug Intoxication

Antiepileptic drug-plasma concentration determinations can assist in evaluating antiepileptic drug intoxication in at least two ways. First, many antiepileptic drugs produce similar toxic symptoms (e.g., drowsiness, ataxia, diplopia). If a patient is taking more than one drug, antiepileptic drug-plasma concentration determinations can determine which drug in the plasma is present in supratherapeutic concentration and is, therefore, presumably responsible for the patient's toxic symptoms. Second, knowledge of a drug's plasma concentration and elimination half-life can enable the physician to make an educated guess as to how long the drug causing intoxication must be withheld before therapy is resumed at a lower dosage.

4. Documentation of Continued Compliance

There is a great tendency for patients whose seizures are controlled to begin omitting some of their medication. One estimate is that patients who are seizure-free omit one pill per day for every 6 months they are seizure-free. Antiepileptic-drug-plasma concentrations should be determined every 6 to 12 months in patients whose seizures are controlled to detect noncompliance and prevent recurrence of seizures.

5. Pregnancy

During pregnancy, multiple pharmacokinetic changes usually result in a net decrease in plasma concentration of antiepileptic drugs (see Chapter 13). Total (protein-bound plus free or non-protein-bound) plasma concentration usually decreases to a greater extent than free plasma concentration. Routine monitoring of free plasma concentration is recommended during pregnancy to ensure adequate antiepileptic effect.

6. Other Diseases

Routine monitoring of antiepileptic drug-plasma concentrations is recommended in the presence of other disease which can alter the absorption, distribution, protein binding, biotransformation, or excretion of antiepileptic drugs. Determination of free plasma concentration is useful in conditions where protein binding may be altered (pregnancy, renal failure, liver failure).

D. Sampling Conditions

Whenever possible, the blood sampling time for individual patients should be standardized to ensure comparable conditions. Ideally, the samples should be taken at the end of the longest interval between doses (usually just before the morning dose of drug). In outpatients, the morning dose can be postponed a couple of hours to ensure this. If the drug-plasma concentration is adequate at this time, it will be adequate throughout the rest of the day. When toxic symptoms of the drug are suspected during the day, it is best to draw the sample at the time of maximal plasma drug level.

The following patient data are necessary for a meaningful evaluation of drug levels: age, weight, sex, diagnosis, indications for analysis, clinical conditions of relevance, all drugs in use with total daily dosages, and sampling time in relation to the last drug intake.

E. Interpretation

1. Causes of Low Plasma Concentration

These include: noncompliance, poor absorption, steady state not reached, change in drug formulation, rapid metabolism, drug interactions, pregnancy, hypoalbuminemia, renal dysfunction, patient taking wrong dose, laboratory error.

2. Causes of High Plasma Concentration

These include: patient taking wrong dose (intentionally or unintentionally), change in drug formulation, drug interactions, hepatic disease, laboratory error.

VIII. DISCONTINUING THERAPY

Uncontrolled seizures and seizures caused by a progressive neurologic illness (e.g., astrocytoma) are indications for continuing antiepileptic drug therapy indefinitely. Antiepileptic drug therapy usually should be maintained for a minimum of 2 to 3 years after diagnosis of epilepsy, even if the patient has no further seizures. When a patient has been free of seizures for 2 to 3 years on antiepileptic drug therapy, the need for continued therapy can be re-evaluated. Risk factors have been identified that help evaluate the likelihood of seizures recurring after medication has been discontinued.

Risk factors for seizure recurrence include: (a) occurrence of many seizures before seizures are controlled; (b) more than one type of partial or generalized seizure; (c) abnormal neurologic examination or low IQ; and (d) failure of EEG to normalize during treatment. The risk of seizure recurrence is approximately 25% in patients without risk factors and > 50% in patients with risk factors. Approximately 80% of seizure recurrences occur within 4 months of beginning to taper drugs, and 90% occur within the first year. Driving and other dangerous activities should be prohibited for at least the first 4 months after starting drug withdrawal.

Each decision must be made on an individual basis. A history of seizure frequency and risk factors must be obtained. A routine EEG is highly useful, and a long-term

EEG recording is sometimes desirable. The probability of recurrent seizures, the consequences of having another seizure, and the benefits of living without medication must be discussed with the patient; the judgment must be weighted by the needs of the individual.

If it is elected to discontinue antiepileptic therapy, medication should be withdrawn slowly. Elimination of one pill per day (or 25% of daily dosage) every five elimination half-lives, is probably the optimal regimen. In general, more rapid tapering of therapy may precipitate seizures, and more prolonged withdrawal probably does not reduce the risk of seizure recurrence. Special caution is required when discontinuing benzodiazepines, especially clonazepam.

IX. MEDICALLY INTRACTABLE EPILEPSY

Many cases of so-called "intractable" epilepsy are caused by improper diagnosis of seizure type (resulting in the use of improper antiepileptic drugs), failure to push the drugs used to the maximal dosage, or failure to use all available antiepileptic drugs. There are some patients, however, who continue to have seizures despite a proper seizure diagnosis and maximal therapy with conventional antiepileptic drugs. Patients with partial seizures should be considered for cortical resection procedures after failure of three antiepileptic drugs to provide adequate control. The efficacy and safety of such procedures in properly selected patients are well-proven (see following). In patients whose seizures are not controlled with conventional drugs and who are not candidates for cortical resection procedures, there are four therapeutic options: (a) less commonly used antiepileptic drugs (Chapter 11); (b) experimental drugs (Chapter 11); (c) experimental surgical procedures (see following); and (d) behavioral therapies [see Wolf (20)]. Such therapies usually are available only at specialized epilepsy centers.

X. SURGERY

While antiepileptic drug therapy is the treatment of choice for most patients with epilepsy, a significant number of patients with seizures respond to surgical treatment. Deciding whether to do a surgical evaluation is dependent upon a clear understanding of the indications and contraindications for epilepsy surgery.

A. Selection of Patients for Referral

1. Indications (See Table 10-4)

Medically intractable seizures is usually defined as persistence of seizures despite trials of three or more antiepileptic drugs, alone or in combination. Each of the drugs should be pushed to maximum tolerated dosage as described earlier.

The *seizures must significantly reduce the quality of life.* In persons with severe physical, mental, or psychiatric handicaps, reducing their seizure frequency may have little impact on overall quality of life. In such persons, the risks and expense of surgery are not justified.

A *localized seizure focus* by EEG or magnetic resonance imaging (MRI) scan suggests the patient will benefit from one of the cortical resection procedures which have a high success rate and low morbidity (see following). However, some patients with multifocal epilepsy can benefit from other surgical procedures (see following).

Biologic predictors of seizure persistence include frequent seizures, early seizure onset, secondary generalization, structural lesion, and abnormal neurologic status. The presence of these predictors suggests the seizures are unlikely to improve with passage of time.

2. Contraindications (See Table 10-4)

Benign, self-limited epilepsy syndromes include benign Rolandic epilepsy and benign focal epilepsy of childhood with occipital spikes. Also the seizures of Landau-Kleffner syndrome typically remit by late adolescence.

In patients with *severe family dysfunction, psychosis, or mental retardation* surgical reduction in seizure frequency seldom results in a significant improvement in quality

TABLE 10-4. Indications and contraindications for epilepsy surgery procedures

Indications	Medically intractable seizures (necessary)
	Seizures significantly reduce quality of life (necessary)
	Localized seizure focus (helpful)
	Biologic predictors of seizure persistence (helpful)
Contraindications	Benign, self-limited epilepsy syndromes
	Neurodegenerative and metabolic disorders
	Noncompliance with medication
	Severe family dysfunction
	Psychosis

of life. The other problems continue to dominate their existence.

3. Timing

A trial of drug at maximum tolerated dosage for 3 to 6 months usually is adequate to determine if it is effective. Trials of three drugs should take 12 to 24 months. If a patient has failed three antiepileptic drugs, epilepsy surgery should be considered immediately for three reasons. First, the longer the patient lives as a disabled epileptic, the more difficult it is to become fully functional after successful epilepsy surgery. Second, there is evidence seizures may cause brain damage and worsen the seizure disorder and neuropsychological handicaps. Third, there is evidence seizures may have adverse effects on the developing brain.

See the review of Duchowny (10) for further details on selection of patients for referral for epilepsy surgery.

B. Presurgical Evaluation

1. Fundamental Concepts

The fundamental concept of surgery in patients with partial epilepsies is to identify the area of seizure onset and determine whether it can be safely resected. While the most important test is the recording of habitual seizures during EEG monitoring, information provided by the history, neurologic examination, neuropsychological evaluation, and neuroimaging (both anatomic and functional), can provide valuable supporting information. While each epilepsy center has its own surgical protocol, there is general agreement that surgery should be performed only when there is concordance of diagnostic studies as to location of the epileptic focus.

An accurate description of the clinical manifestations of spontaneous seizures is probably the most important piece of clinical information derived from the history. While observers usually concentrate on the most dramatic portion of the seizure, it is important to closely question eye witnesses about the initial phases of the seizure. An aura, no matter how brief, often provides considerable localizing information. In infantile spasms, eye deviation or focal twitching, prior to the spasm, provides information that the seizure began focally. Likewise, a history of asymmetries of strength postically, even if subtle, may provide important localization findings as to seizure onset.

With the widespread use of computerized tomography (CT) and MRI, the value of the neurologic examination has been reduced. However, asymmetries of strength or reflexes may provide evidence of focal pathology, even in the face of normal neuroimaging.

2. Imaging Studies

High-quality MRI is essential in the evaluation of a patient undergoing a surgical evaluation. The MRI is particularly valuable in detecting mesial temporal sclerosis or cerebral dysgenesis (see Chapter 3). Computer-assisted volume analysis of the temporal lobes may detect asymmetries that are not readily apparent on visual analysis of the scan. Focal abnormalities on the MRI, when corresponding to seizure onset on EEG, provides powerful localizing information. In general, patients with focal abnormalities on MRI have a more favorable prognosis for successful surgery than patients with normal MRI.

Single photon emission computed tomographic (SPECT) and positron emission tomography (PET) are becoming increasingly used in the evaluation of patients with intractable epilepsy. Central to the use of SPECT in the localization of the epileptic foci are the observations that ictal hyperperfusion occurs at the site of the epileptic focus, while on the interictal scan hypofusion is usually seen. There is increasing evidence that the ictal scan is superior to the interictal scan in the localization of the epileptic focus.

Like SPECT, PET scanning is a noninvasive functional imaging test that has been used to evaluate cerebral metabolic rates. While many agents have been labeled with positron-emitters, 2-deoxy-2[^{18}F]fluoro-D-glucose (FDG) has been the agent most commonly used in epilepsy. The interictal scan typically demonstrates hypometabolism, while a scan obtained during a seizure demonstrates hypermetabolism. Positron emission tomography scanning has been found to be a useful adjunctive test in the evaluation of both children and adults with epilepsy. The PET may be superior to MRI in localizing focal areas of cortical dysplasia and other structural abnormalities corresponding to surface-EEG localization of epileptogenic regions. In the hands of experienced investigators, the PET may eliminate or reduce the need for invasive monitoring. Unfortunately, PET scans are available in only a few centers.

3. Neuropsychological Studies

Like the neurologic examination, the neuropsychological evaluation can provide useful localizing information. The focal area where a seizure begins often also has disturbed neuropsychological function. For example, patients with seizures arising in the dominant temporal lobe may have deficits in verbal memory or language acquisition, while deficits in visuospatial memory suggest seizure onset in the nondominant temporal lobe. Significant deficits in both, suggest bilateral temporal lobe damage and would make surgical resection of one temporal lobe risky (see following).

The *intracarotid amobarbital test ("Wada test")* involves performance of neuropsychological testing after a region of the brain has been inactivated with amobarbital delivered through selective intracarotid injection. This injection mimics the effect of surgical removal of the region and allows one to determine if the remaining structures can carry out the tasks being studied. Such testing is important if removal of mesial temporal structures is being considered. Memory requires at least one functioning mesial temporal area. Mesial temporal damage is sometimes bilateral. Removal of one mesial temporal area in a patient with bilateral mesial temporal damage may leave the patient with severe memory deficits. Preoperative testing allows one to know the remaining mesial temporal area can sustain memory function. The intracarotid amobarbital test is also routinely used to determine the dominant hemisphere for language. This information assists in planning the extent of surgery which can be safely performed.

4. EEG

Despite the development of newer imaging techniques, EEG investigation remains the cornerstone for localization of the epileptic foci. Both interictal and ictal epileptiform activity are used in the localization of the epileptic zone. In the early years of epilepsy surgery, interictal discharges recorded with scalp electrodes were the primary means for localization. However, interictal discharges on scalp recording are absent in some patients, poorly localized or bilaterally independent in others, and occasionally falsely localizing. Thus, interictal discharges are rarely used as the *sole* means of localization. The onset of an electroencephalographic seizure is considered the most reliable of the localizing signs. However, there are a number of problems that may occur which limit the usefulness of the ictal EEG. Artifacts may obscure the electro-cephalographic seizure, seizures may be poorly localized, or the electroencephalographic seizures may follow the onset of the clinical seizure.

In instances where seizures can not be well-localized using surface electrodes, or when the SPECT, PET, MRI, or neuropsychological data is not concordant with the EEG findings, intracranial electrodes are typically used. While a variety of different types of intracranial electrodes have been used, the most common types are depth, subdural, and epidural. Depth electrodes consist of thin wires with multiple EEG-recording contacts. Depth electrodes are implanted stereotaxically and can be implanted into a variety of cerebral structures; subdural electrodes are placed over the surface of the brain. Depth electrodes allow accurate recordings from structures located at a distance from the surface, and are particularly valuable when the clinician suspects the seizures are arising from the amygdala or hippocampus.

Subdural or epidural electrodes consist of strips or grids of electrodes imbedded into a thin sheet of plastic. The plastic sheet is quite pliable and is easily inserted into the subdural or epidural space. Subdural or epidural electrodes grids may be helpful in planning a safe, effective resection for patients with an epileptogenic region near functional cortex, since the clinician can electrically stimulate the electrodes to map functional cortex. While subdural electrodes grids may be slipped under the edges of the open craniotomy (including under the temporal or frontal lobe or in the interhemispheric fissure), epidural electrode grids can cover just the exposed area. In addition, cortical stimulation with epidural electrodes may cause pain because of stimulation of meningeal nerve fibers.

As electrodes become more invasive, they tend to provide more detailed and precisely localized information, at the expense of more limited sampling. The most invasive techniques, such as depth electrodes and epidural or subdural grids, are helpful in answering specific neurophysiological questions concerning a restricted cortical area; but they are less helpful to explore more widespread localization problems between large cortical areas. Therefore, these techniques should be reserved for cases where basic localization problems have already been resolved by scalp EEG and other diagnostic studies.

C. Surgical Procedures (See Table 10-5)

1. Temporal Lobe Seizures

Temporal lobe resection is an effective procedure in selected children and adults with uncontrolled complex partial seizures. The surgical approach varies from center to center. Some centers advocate resections where the amount of tissue removed is determined by intraoperative corticography and stimulation studies. The resection may be limited, consisting only of an amygdalohippocampectomy. Other centers use an "en bloc" resection in which the anterior temporal lobe is removed in one piece. There are no studies convincingly demonstrating better results of one method over the other.

While there are differences from center to center, patients undergoing surgical resection of the temporal lobe have a 70% to 80% chance of either becoming seizure-free or having significant improvement.

2. Nontemporal Lobe Seizures

Temporal lobectomy is the most frequent type of epilepsy surgery among patients overall, but extratemporal resection is becoming more common. Locating a seizure focus in nontemporal lobe structures is more difficult than in the temporal lobe, unless the patient has a structural lesion. This is particularly difficult when the seizures are suspected to arise from the frontal lobe. The large surface of the frontal lobe, as well as anatomic structures like the mesial and orbital regions that are far removed from the recording electrodes, makes it difficult to localize either interictal or ictal EEG abnormalities. Focal EEG seizures may also arise in a "silent" region of the frontal lobe producing clinical symptomatology only after a seizure spreads to neighboring frontal lobe structures or to the temporal lobe.

The task is made even more complicated by the existence of a functional network of pathways permitting spread of discharges within and outside the frontal lobes. The bidirectional spread of epileptic discharges through the uncinate fasciculus and the cingulate gyrus in seizures arising from the frontal lobe, may be falsely localized to the temporal lobe and vice versa. Because of this difficulty in localizing abnormalities, there is poorer electro-clinical correlation of ictal events in the frontal lobe than elsewhere. Most patients with frontal lobe seizures that do not have structural lesions on MRI require invasive electrode monitoring.

TABLE 10-5. Summary of surgical procedures for patients with medically intractable seizures

Procedure	Seizure type	EEG	Risks	Benefits
Temporal lobectomy	Partial[a] ± 2nd general[b]	Interictal:temporal or frontal spikes, sharp waves.Ictal:Initially discharges (spikes, sharp waves,beta, or rhythmic slowing) from temporal lobe, may then spread.	Quadrantanopic field deficit; . cerebrovascular. accident; 3rd nerve palsy.	Seizure control or significant reduction of seizures
Nontemporal resections	Partial[a] ± 2nd general[b]	Interictal: focal spikes/sharp waves, occasional generalized spike waves. Ictal: Focal spikes, beta activity, rapid spikes, spike-wave, polyspike-wave	Dependent on surgical site weakness; visual field cut	Seizure control or significant reduction in seizures; improved development
Corpus callostomy	Partial[a] ± 2nd general[b] tonic, atonic, "drop" attacks	Interictal: Mutifocal spikes/sharp waves, generalized spike-wave, polyspike-wave. Ictal: Rapid spikes, spike-wave, polyspike-wave	Disconnection	Reduction in "drop" and generalized seizures; rarely do seizures totally remit
Hemisperectomy	Unilateral partial[a] ± 2nd general seizure[b], hemiparesis	Interictal: Preponderance of lateralized EEG discharges over involved hemisphere; may have bilateral spikes. Ictal: Lateralized onset to seizure over involved hemisphere.	Hemiparesis; homonymous; hemianopsia	Seizure control; improved behavioral and cognitive state

[a]Simple or complex partial seizures.
[b]Secondarily generalized tonic-clonic seizures.

The incidence of excellent outcome with patients seizure-free or with a significant reduction in seizure after extratemporal resection is only roughly 50%. However, with improving anatomic and functional neuroimaging, it is likely that these statistics will improve.

3. Hemispherectomy

The removal of all or most of one hemisphere is one of the most drastic, yet effective, means to treat seizures. The procedure is typically used in patients with severe unilateral motor seizures who already have a hemiparesis and nonfunctional hand. Patients with Rasmussen's encephalitis and Sturge-Weber syndrome are frequently candidates for this type of surgery. In addition, patients with hemimegalencephaly and other disorders of cerebral dysgenesis, cerebral infarctions, and trauma may also benefit from the surgery.

The presurgical evaluation must establish that the patient is not a candidate for a more restricted surgical resection. While bilateral interictal spikes are common in patients with unilateral hemisphere pathology, determination that the seizures begin unilaterally is essential. However, this may be difficult to establish in patients with severe atrophy of the hemisphere, when only surface EEG monitoring is performed, since the ictal discharges may not propagate well to the surface of the head. In these cases, the clinical features of the seizures and functional neuroimaging can be useful in lateralizing the epileptic focus.

The response to the procedure is gratifying with over three-quarters of the patients having a favorable outcome following the procedure. Because of late complications including superficial hemosiderosis with obstructive hydrocephalus, bleeding into the hemispherectomy cavity, or fatal brain-stem shift, surgeons have been performing modified hemispherectomies that isolate, but do not remove, the frontal and occipital poles or hemicortectomy.

4. Corpus Callosotomy

In some patients, despite extensive evaluations, a focus cannot be identified. In others, presurgical evaluation will detect more than one focus. These patients may benefit from a corpus callosotomy. In this procedure, epileptic tissue is not removed but the spread of the seizures altered.

At the present time there are no firm criteria that can be used to predict which patient will benefit from corpus callosotomy. Factors that have been associated with favorable outcomes by some, but not all investigators, have included normal intelligence, focal EEG abnormalities, focal abnormalities on the CT or MRI scan, the presence of generalized tonic-clonic, tonic, and atonic seizures and hemiparesis. The procedure is usually reserved for patients with very frequent seizures, particularly "drop" attacks (atonic and tonic seizures).

Although complications from the corpus callosotomy are relatively few, the procedure is not without risk. Infection and infarction have occurred following the procedure and, rarely, patients may die. A disconnection syndrome has been described following the callosotomy. Patients may have difficulties with speech and motor functioning for days to weeks following the surgery. There may be decreased spontaneity of speech, which may be as severe as complete mutism or as mild as a slowness in initiating speech. In addition, variable degrees of paresis of the nondominant leg, forced grasping of the nondominant hand, and incontinence are present. These deficits usually improve with speech and physical therapy. However, there have been reports of permanent language disturbances after isolated anterior, posterior, or complete callosotomy; but only in patients with mixed cerebral dominance. When the hemisphere with language dominance is not the hemisphere controlling handedness, language deficits are more likely to develop. In these patients, a prior injury to the dominant hemisphere may cause transfer of some expressive language to the contralateral hemisphere, without changing the preferred hand.

Table 10-5 is a summary table for common epilepsy surgical procedures.

D. Special Considerations in Children

While many of the principles applied to adult patients with epilepsy are relevant to children with medically intractable seizures, epilepsy surgery in children presents a number of unique challenges and differences from adults. Some seizure disorders in children are catastrophic. In disorders such as infantile spasms or Sturge-Weber syndrome, the clinician is often faced not only with frequent, medically intractable seizures but a "plateauing" or even decline in development. Children may have major neurologic impairment from the recurrent seizures or effects of antiepileptic drugs during the crucial early years of learning. Removing the focal brain abnormality, theoretically, will allow the remainder of the brain to develop free of the undesirable influences of the abnormal epileptic tissue and antiepileptic drug therapy.

However, many childhood seizure disorders remit spontaneously, and performing surgery on a child who will eventually go into remission is inappropriate. While it is not always possible to know the natural course of the seizure disorder, surgery should not be considered unless there is a high likelihood that remission is not going to occur. It should also be remembered that while epilepsy surgery offers hope to a number of children with severe epilepsy, surgery is certainly not risk-free. The risk of creating a permanent deficit must be balanced with the likelihood that the surgery will eliminate or significantly reduce the frequency of the seizures.

REFERENCES

1. Adelson PD, Black P McL. Surgical treatment of epilepsy in children. Neurosurgery Clinics of North America, Vol. 6, 1995.
2. American Academy of Neurology Quality Standards Subcommittee. Practice parameter: a guideline for discontinuing antiepileptic drugs in seizure-free patients—summary statement. *Neurology* 1996;46: 600–602.
3. Beghi E, Berg AT, Hauser WA. Treatment of single seizures. In: Engel J, Pedley TA, eds. *Epilepsy: a comprehensive textbook*. Philadelphia: Lippincott–Raven, 1997.
4. Brodie MJ, Dichter MA. Antiepileptic drugs. *N Engl J Med* 1996;334:168–175.
5. Browne TR. Clinical pharmacology and pharmacokinetics of antiepileptic drugs. In: Chokroverty S, ed. *Modern management of epilepsy*. Boston: Butterworth-Heinemann, 1996.
6. Commission on Antiepileptic Drugs of International League Against Epilepsy. Guidelines for therapeutic monitoring of antiepileptic drugs. *Epilepsia* 1993;34: 585–587.
7. Dichter MA, Brodie MJ. New antiepileptic drugs. *N Engl J Med* 1996;334:1583–1590.
8. Engel J, Pedley TA, eds. *Epilepsy: a comprehensive textbook*. Philadelphia: Lippincott–Raven, 1997, Chapters 94–127, 160–179.
9. Engel J. Surgery for seizures. *N Engl J Med* 1996; 334:647–652.

10. Duchowny M. Identification of surgical candidates and timing of operation: an overview. In: Wyllie E, ed. *The treatment of epilepsy: principles and practice,* 2nd ed. Baltimore: Williams and Wilkins, 1997.

11. Hauser WA. The natural history of seizures. In: Wyllie E. ed. *The treatment of epilepsy: principles and practice,* 2nd ed. Baltimore: Williams and Wilkins, 1997.

12. Hernandez TD, Naritoku DK. Seizures, epilepsy, and functional recovery after brain surgery. *Neurology* 1997;48:1383–1388.

13. Levy RH, Bourgeois B. Drug–drug interactions. In: Engel J, Pedley TA, eds. *Epilepsy: a comprehensive textbook.* Philadelphia: Lippincott–Raven, 1997.

14. Mattson RH. Antiepileptic drug monitoring: a reappraisal. *Epilepsia* 1995;36(suppl 5):S22–S29.

15. Mattson RH. Selection of antiepileptic drug therapy. In: Levy RH, Mattson RH, Meldrum BS, eds. *Antiepileptic drugs*, 4th ed. New York: Raven Press, 1995.

16. Moshe SL, Pellock JM, Salon MCL. *The Parke Davis manual on epilepsy: useful tips that help you get the best out of life.* New York: RSF Group, 1993 (includes discussion of many psychosocial topics).

17. Porter RJ. How to use antiepileptic drugs. In: Levy RH, Mattson RH, Meldrum BS, eds. *Antiepileptic drugs*, 4th ed. New York: Raven Press, 1995 (includes discussion of medically intractable epilepsy).

18. Tatro DS. *Drug interactions facts.* St. Louis: Facts and Comparisons, 1997.

19. Theodore W, Porter RJ. *Epilepsy: 100 Elementary Principles*, 2nd ed. London: WB Saunders, 1995.

20. Wolf P. Behavioral therapy. In: Engel J, Pedley TA, eds. *Epilepsy: a comprehensive textbook.* Philadelphia: Lippincott–Raven, 1997.

21. Wyllie E. ed. *The treatment of epilepsy: principles and practice,* 2nd ed. Baltimore: Williams and Wilkins, 1997, Chapters 49–60, 74–88.

ANTIEPILEPTIC DRUGS

This chapter will review the mechanisms of action, indications, pharmacokinetics and clinical usage of the drugs commonly used to treat epilepsy (Tables 11-1, 11-2, and 11-3). The experimental antiepileptic drug vigabatrin will also be discussed because it may be approved by the United States Food and Drug Administration (FDA) shortly after this book is published. Drugs will be reviewed in alphabetical order. Pharmacological principles of drug administration, drugs of choice for various seizure types, and discontinuing antiepileptic drug therapy are reviewed in Chapter 10.

I. MECHANISM OF ACTION

Marketed antiepileptic drugs work by varying combinations of mechanisms described further on. The specific mechanism(s) of action of specific, marketed antiepileptic drugs are listed in Table 11-1.

A. Sodium Currents

The firing of an action potential by an axon requires passage of sodium into the axon through sodium channels. Sodium channels exist in three states: (a) resting (able to allow passage of sodium); (b) active (allowing passage of sodium); and (c) inactive (not allowing passage of sodium). After activation, a percentage of sodium channels become inactivated for a period of time. With repetitive axonal firing, enough sodium channels become inactivated that the axon can no longer propagate an action potential. Some antiepileptic drugs stabilize the inactive form of the sodium channel, preventing its return to the active state. This, in turn, prevents sustained repetitive firing of the axon.

B. GABA$_A$ Receptor Currents

Attachment of gamma-aminobutyric acid (GABA) to GABA$_A$ receptors facilitates the passage of chloride ions through chloride channels into cells. Chloride ions are negatively charged. Their passage into the cell makes the resting membrane potential more negative inside the cell and makes it more difficult for the cell to depolarize. Some antiepileptic drugs are agonists of this type of GABA-mediated chloride conductance.

TABLE 11-1. Mechanism(s) of action and pharmacokinetics of antiepileptic drugs

Drug	Mechanism of action[a]	Elimination half-life in children (hr)	Elimination half-life in adults (hr)	Time to steady state plasma concentration (days)	Protein binding (%)
Carbamazepine (Tegretol)	A	14–27 (children) 8—28 (neonates)	14–27	3–4	66–89
Clonazepam (Klonopin)	A,B	20–40	20–40	—	86
Ethosuximide (Zarontin)	C	20–60	20—60	7–10	0
Gabapentin (Neurontin)	E	—	5–7	—	0
Lamotrigine (Lamoctal)	A,D	—	See text	—	55
Phenobarbital	A,B	37–73	40–136	12–21	40–60
Phenytoin (Dilantin)	A	5–14 (children) 10–60 (neonates)	12–36	7–28	69–96
Primidone (Mysoline)	A,B	5–11	6–18	4–7	0
Topiramate (Topamax)	A,B,D	—	20–30, 12–15[b]	—	15
Valproic Acid (Depakene, Depakote)	A,B	8–15	6–15	1–2	80–95

[a]A, sodium currents; B, GABA$_A$ receptor currents; C, T-calcium currents; D, glutamate receptor antagonist; E, unknown. See Section I of this chapter for discussion.

[b]In the presence of enzyme-inducing drugs such as carbamazepine, phenobarbital, or primidone.

TABLE 11-2. Usual pediatric dosages of antiepileptic drugs

Drug	Starting dose (mg/day)	Dosing regimen	Dose escalation rate (in daily dose/time interval)	Maintenance dose (mg/day)	Therapeutic range of plasma concentration (μg/ml)[a]
Carbamazepine (Tegretol)	<6yr: 10–15mg/kg 6–12 yr: 100 mg b.i.d.	t.i.d.	<6 yr: 5 mg/kg/1 week >6 yr: 100–200 mg/1 week	10–30 mg/kg/day	4–12
Clonzaepam (Klonopin)	<10 yr: or <30 kg: 0.01–0.3 mg/kg/day >10 yr: 1–1.5 mg/day	t.i.d.–q.i.d.	<10 yr: 0.02 mg/kg/1 wk >10 yr: 0.5 mg/1 wk	0.1–0.3 mg/kg/day	0.02–0.08
Ethosuximide (Zarontin)	<6 yr: 10–15 mg/kg not to exceed 250 mg >6 yr: 250 mg/day	t.i.d.–q.i.d.	125–250 mg/1 week	15–40 mg/kg/day	120
Gabapentin (Neurontin)	10 mg/kg/day	t.i.d.	300 mg/1 day	30–60 mg/kg (Not yet established)	Not established
Lamotrigine (Lamictal)	25 mg/day. If on valproic acid/Divalroex sodium: 12.5 mg q.o.d.	b.i.d.	25mg/week	Monotherapy:10 mg/day If on enzyme inducer:[b] 15 mg/kg/day If on enzyme inhibitor:[c] 5 mg/kg/day	Not established
Phenobarbital	<1 yr: 3–5mg/kg >1 yr: 2–4 mg/kg	b.i.d.–q.d.	1–2mg/kg/2 weeks	<1 yr: 3–5 mg/kg >1 yr: 2–4 mg/kg	10–40
Phenytoin (Dilantin)	5 mg/kg/day	b.i.d.	1–2 mg/kg/2 weeks	5–8 mg/kg/day	10–25
Primidone (Mysoline)	<6 yr: 50 mg/day >12 yr: 100 mg/day	q.i.d.–t.i.d.	25–50 mg/2 weeks	12–25 mg/kg/day	5–12
Topiramate (Topamax)	1 mg/kg/day	b.i.d.	1 mg/kg/week	5–10 mg/kg/day	not established
Valproic Acid (Depakene) Divalporex sodium (Depakote)	15–20 mg/kg/day	Valproic acid q.i.d.–t.i.d. Divalproex sodium b.i.d.	5–10 mg/kg/day	30–80 mg/kg/day	50–150

[a]See Appendix I for conversion to molar units. [b]Carbamazepine, phenobarbital, phenytoin, primidone. [c]Valproic acid, divalproex sodium.

TABLE 11-3. Usual adult dosages of antiepileptic drugs (16 years and older)

Drug	Starting dose (mg/day)	Dosing regimen	Escalation rate (in daily dose/time interval)	Maintenance dose (mg/day)	Maximum dose (mg/day)	Therapeutic range of plasma concentration (µg/ml)[a]
Carbamazepine (Tegretol)	200	Tegretol-XR b.i.d.; other forms t.i.d.	200/1 week	600–1,200	1,600	4–12
Clonazepam (Klonapin)	1.5	t.i.d.	0.5/4 days	2–6	20	0.02–0.08
Ethosuximide (Zarontin)	500	t.i.d.	250/1 week	1,000–2,000		40–120
Gabapentin (Neurontin)	300	t.i.d.	300/daily	900–3,600		Not established
Lamotrigine (Lamictal)	See text	b.i.d.	See text	See text	700	Not established
Phenobarbital	90	q.d.[b]	30/4 weeks	90–120	—	10–40
Phenytoin (Dilantin)	300	q.d.[b]	30–100[c]/4 weeks	300–500	—	10–40
Primidone (Mysoline)	100–125	t.i.d.	See text	750–1,000	2,000	5–12
Topiramate (Topamax)	50	b.i.d.	See text	200–400	1,600	Not established
Valproic acid (Depakene) (Depakote)	1,000	Valproic acid t.i.d.; Divalproex sodium b.i.d.	250/1 week	1,000–3,000	4,000 (60 mg/kg/day)	50–150

[a]See Appendix I for conversion to molar units.
[b]Once daily drugs are usually given at bedtime to avoid toxicity associated with peak plasma concentrations.
[c]Increments of 100 mg/day if plasma concentration below 10 µg/ml. Increments of 30–50 mg/day if plasma concentration above 10 µg/ml.

C. T-Calcium Currents

T-calcium currents are one of three different voltage-dependent calcium currents (L,N,T) known to exist in the human brain. T-calcium currents are small, rapidly inactivated currents that act as pacemakers for normal rhythmic brain activity, especially in the thalamus. T-calcium currents also appear to have an important role in pacing the three per second spike-wave activity of absence seizures (but not other seizure types). Drugs inhibiting T-calcium currents specifically inhibit absence seizures.

D. Glutamate Receptor Antagonists

Excitation in the human nervous system is produced principally by binding of the excitory amino acid glutamate to three types of ionotropic glutamate receptors: NMDA, AMPA, and kainate. Binding of glutamate to these receptors facilitates passage of calcium and sodium into the cell and potassium out of the cell. The net effect is reduction of the negative resting-membrane potential, making the cell less electrically stable. Some antiepileptic drugs act by antagonism of one or more types of glutamate receptor.

II. CARBAMAZEPINE (TEGRETOL)

A. Mechanism of Action

See Section I and Table 11-1.

B. Indications, Advantages, and Disadvantages

Carbamazepine is indicated as initial or adjunctive therapy for complex partial and tonic-clonic seizures. Carbamazepine was found to be one of the two safest and most effective drugs for these seizure types in comparative studies of older drugs (phenytoin is the other). It is relatively nonsedating (sedation is mild and similar to that of phenytoin) and does not have the cosmetic side effects of phenytoin.

A loading dose of carbamazepine cannot be administered by any route. The drug must be given in divided doses. Carbamazepine must be started at a low dose, and the dosage must be built up over time. Carbamazepine may exacerbate absence seizures in some patients. There is an increased risk of spina bifida in infants born to mothers taking carbamazepine during pregnancy.

C. Pharmacokinetics (See Table 11-1)

Approximately 75% to 85% of an orally administered dose of brand-name Tegretol, 200 mg tablets, is slowly absorbed after oral administration. The bioavailability of generic carbamazepine is usually less than that of brand-name Tegretol. Carbamazepine is 70% to 80% protein-bound. Carbamazepine is metabolized by the liver into 32 or more metabolites, some of which (especially epoxide) possess antiepileptic activity. Carbamazepine biotransformation exhibits time-dependent pharmacokinetics (self-induction), which means that the plasma concentration may fall unexpectedly during the first 2 months of administration when self-induction occurs.

D. Usual Pediatric and Adult Dosages

See Tables 11-2 and 11-3.

E. Formulations

Carbamazepine is marketed as standard 200 mg tablets (both generic and as the brand name Tegretol) as well as 200 mg Tegretol XR tablets.

Tegretol XR is a constant-release carbamazepine preparation using osmotic pump-tablet technology. Twice-daily dosing with the XR formulation produces mean plasma concentrations similar to those obtained with 3-times-daily administration of standard carbamazepine tablets with less peak-to-trough variability. This reduces the toxicity associated with high peak values and the breakthrough seizures associated with low trough values. Many experts believe that the Tegretol XR formulation is the carbamazepine formulation of choice for most adults. Carbamazepine is also formulated in 100 mg chewable tablets and suspension (100 mg/5 cc) for pediatric usage.

F. Toxicity

Local toxicity consists of gastric irritability that is usually managed by taking the drug after meals. Common dose-related toxicity includes diplopia or blurred vision, dizziness, drowsiness, ataxia, and headache. At high plasma concentrations, the following may occur: tremor, dystonia, chorea, depression, irritability, psychosis, convulsions, water retention (inappropriate antidiuretic-hormone-like syndrome), congestive heart failure, and cardiac arrhythmias.

Idiosyncratic toxicities are rash (common) and, more rarely, anemia, agranulocytosis, leukopenia, thrombocytopenia, hypersensitivity syndrome (dermatitis, eosino-philia, lymphadenopathy, splenomegaly), and cholestatic and hepatocellular jaundice. The rate of fatal idiosyncratic reactions with carbamazepine is estimated currently at 1 in 100,000 to 200,000 patients. Although this factor is a matter of concern, this risk is in a range similar to other commonly used drugs, such as penicillin.

G. Drug Interactions

Adding carbamazepine may increase the plasma concentration of phenytoin and lower the plasma concentrations of felbamate, lamotrigine, oral contraceptives, theophylline, and valproic acid. Propoxyphene, erythromycin, chloramphenicol, isoniazid, verapamil, and cimetidine may elevate the plasma carbamazepine concentration, whereas phenobarbital, phenytoin, felbamate, and primidone may lower the plasma-carbamazepine concentration. Adding lamotrigine to carbamazepine may enhance the usual neurotoxic side effects of carbamazepine.

H. Disease States

Carbamazepine may precipitate or enhance congestive heart failure. Its use should be avoided in this setting or in cases in which major arrhythmias are a concern. Plasma concentrations and potential toxicity need to be closely watched if the drug is used in patients with renal or hepatic disease.

I. Pregnancy

In common with several other antiepileptic drugs, there is a 2% to 3% increase in fetal epilepsy syndrome in infants born to mothers taking carbamazepine. In addition, there is a 1% risk of spina bifida (vs. 1 in 1,500 in the normal population) in infants born to mothers taking carbamazepine.

III. CLONAZEPAM (KLONOPIN)

A. Mechanism of Action

See Section I and Table 11-1.

B. Indications, Advantages, and Disadvantages

Clonazepam is the third-choice drug for absence seizures because disabling side effects (drowsiness, ataxia, behavior disturbance), and development of tolerance to the antiepileptic effect of the drug, are more common with clonazepam than with ethosuximide or valproic acid. Clonazepam is also indicated as initial or adjunctive therapy for atypical absence, atonic, and myoclonic seizures.

C. Pharmacokinetics (see Table 11-1)
Clonazepam appears to be well-absorbed by the alimentary tract. It is 47% protein-bound. Extensive biotransformation takes place, and less than 0.5% is recovered from the urine as clonazepam.

D. Usual Pediatric and Adult Doses
See Tables 11-2 and 11-3.

E. Formulations
Tablet sizes include 0.5, 1.0, and 2.0 mg.

F. Toxicity
Dose-related toxicity includes drowsiness, ataxia, behavioral change (irritability, depression, psychosis), dysarthria, and diplopia. Idiosyncratic toxicity commonly includes skin rash and, rarely, hair loss, anemia, leukopenia, and thrombocytopenia.

G. Drug Interactions
Phenobarbital may lower the clonazepam plasma concentration. Concurrent use of amphetamines and methylphenidate may cause central nervous system (CNS) depression and respiratory irregularities. Depressant effects may also be enhanced by alcohol, antianxiety and antipsychotic drugs, antidepressants, and other antiepileptic drugs. Concurrent use of valproic acid has, in some individuals, been associated with the development of absence status epilepticus.

H. Disease States
Renal disease is unlikely to affect the elimination of clonazepam, but liver disease may require a decrease in dosage.

I. Pregnancy
There are no adequate studies on clonazepam in pregnant women.

IV. ETHOSUXIMIDE (ZARONTIN)

A. Mechanism of Action
See Section I and Table 11-1.

B. Indications, Advantages, and Disadvantages
Ethosuximide is the drug of first choice for patients with only absence seizures because it is extremely effective, and most patients experience little or no side effects during chronic administration. The common side effects of ethosuximide, gastrointestinal upset, and drowsiness, tend to occur early in therapy and then diminish as tolerance develops. The drug seldom causes behavioral or cognitive disturbances. Approximately 1% to 7% of patients taking ethosuximide develop leukopenia, which is reversible if detected early. Ethosuximide is ineffective against tonic-clonic and myoclonic seizures, which sometimes accompany absence seizures.

C. Pharmacokinetics (see Table 11-1)
Ethosuximide is readily and, almost completely, absorbed in the alimentary tract. There is little or no binding to serum proteins. The drug is transformed in the liver to either a ketone or an alcohol metabolite, which is then excreted with or without glucuronide conjugation.

D. Usual Pediatric and Adult Dosage
See Tables 11-2 and 11-3.

E. Formulations
Ethosuximide is available as a 250 mg capsule or as a syrup (250 mg/5 cc).

F. Toxicity
Local toxicity includes gastric irritation, anorexia, nausea, and vomiting. Dose-related toxicity includes drowsiness, dizziness, and headache. Idiosyncratic toxicity commonly includes rash and leukopenia and, very rarely, pancytopenia, agranulocytosis, aplastic anemia, psychosis, systemic lupus erythematosus (SLE), and Parkinsonian changes.

G. Drug Interactions
There are no known drug interactions of clinical significance.

H. Disease States
Renal and hepatic disorders do not appear to pose major problems for enhanced toxicity of ethosuximide.

I. Pregnancy
There are no adequate studies on ethosuximide in pregnant women.

V. GABAPENTIN (NEURONTIN)

A. Mechanism of Action
The mechanism of action of gabapentin is not firmly established. Gabapentin is not an agonist of the GABA$_A$ receptor. Gabapentin may facilitate release of GABA at times of excessive rates of neuronal firing.

B. Indications, Advantages, and Disadvantages
Gabapentin is indicated as adjunctive therapy for adults with partial seizures (with or without secondary generalization) which are not controlled with first-choice drugs, such as carbamazepine or phenytoin. The six drugs used for this indication are compared in Table 10-2. Gabapentin has no serious toxicity, minimal dose-dependent toxicity, and no drug interactions. There is no need to monitor laboratory values. Gabapentin appears to be a particularly good drug in the elderly because of its low incidence of neurotropic side effects and absence of drug interactions.

A 3 times a day dosing regimen is required, and gabapentin cannot be given as a loading dose. Parenteral administration is not possible. Gabapentin is more expensive than older drugs.

Gabapentin may be approved by the FDA for initial therapy of partial seizures shortly after this book is published. Consult package insert for details.

C. Pharmacokinetics (See Table 11-1)
Gabapentin has a bioavailability of approximately 60% at low doses. At higher doses bioavailability decreases, because gabapentin is absorbed through the saturatable L-amino-acid transport system in the proximal small intestine. Gabapentin is less than 3% protein-bound. The drug is eliminated by renal excretion as unchanged gabapentin. Gabapentin is not appreciably metabolized in humans. The gabapentin elimination half-life is 5 to 7 hr and is not affected by dose or other drugs. A therapeu-

tic range for gabapentin plasma concentration has not been established.

D. Usual Pediatric and Adult Dosage (see Tables 11-2 and 11-3)

Early experience indicated that daily doses of 900–1,800 mg are effective and well-tolerated when gabapentin is used as add-on therapy for refractory partial or tonic-clonic seizures in adults. More recent experience indicates that higher doses up to 3,600 mg per day are usually well-tolerated and produce better seizure control in some patients. The initial dose is 300 mg at bedtime. The dosage may be increased to 300 mg twice daily on day 2, and 300 mg thrice daily on day 3. Further increases may be made in increments of 300 or 400 mg per day as needed, with a 3 times a day regimen. The maximum time between doses should not exceed 12 hr.

E. Formulation

Gabapentin is formulated as 100, 300, and 400 mg capsules.

F. Toxicity and Drug Interactions

No unique side effects have been identified as presumably caused by gabapentin. A minority of patients experience one or more of the following CNS side effects: drowsiness and fatigue, dizziness, ataxia, and diplopia. No idiosyncratic or long-term toxicity has been demonstrated. There are no known drug interactions.

G. Disease States

The clearance of gabapentin is reduced in patients with reduced renal function, including the elderly. Consult the package insert for dosage instructions when renal function is reduced.

H. Pregnancy

There are no adequate studies on gabapentin in pregnant women.

VI. LAMOTRIGINE (LAMICTAL)

A. Mechanism of Action

See Section I and Table 11-1.

B. Indications, Advantages, and Disadvantages

Lamotrigine is indicated as adjunctive therapy for adults with partial seizures which are not controlled with first-choice drugs, such as carbamazepine or phenytoin. The six drugs used for this indication are compared in Table 10-2. Lamotrigine has minimal dose-dependent toxicity, and there is no need to monitor laboratory values. Rash, occasionally, with Stevens-Johnson syndrome, is a recognized side effect and is a significant concern, especially when using the drug in children. Lamotrigine cannot be given as a loading dose, and parenteral administration is not possible. There are some modest drug interactions. Lamotrigine is more expensive than older drugs.

C. Pharmacokinetics (See Table 11-1)

Lamotrigine is rapidly and completely absorbed following oral administration. Protein binding is 55%. Lamotrigine undergoes hepatic metabolism and is excreted primarily as the 2-*N*-glucuronide metabolite. The elimination half-life of lamotrigine is 30 hr when taken alone, and this value does not change with chronic administration. Co-administration with carbamazepine, phenytoin, or phenobarbital reduces the elimination half-life to 15 hours (co-administration with valproic acid increases the elimination half-life of lamotrigine to 60 hours or more). A therapeutic range for lamotrigine-plasma concentration has not been established.

D. Usual Pediatric and Adult Dosages (See Tables 11-2 and 11-3)

In adults taking enzyme-inducing antiepileptic drugs (carbamazepine, phenobarbital, phenytoin, primidone) and no valproic acid, the starting dosage of lamotrigine is 50 mg once daily for weeks 1 and 2. The dosage is escalated to 50 mg twice per day for weeks 3 and 4. Further adjustments are made at the rate of 100 mg/day every week. The usual maintenance dose is 300 to 500 mg/day in two divided doses.

In adults taking enzyme-inducing antiepileptic drugs and valproic acid, the starting dosage of lamotrigine is 25 mg every other day for weeks 1 and 2. The dosage is escalated to 25 mg once daily for weeks 3 and 4. Further adjustments are made at the rate of 25 to 50 mg/day every 1 or 2 weeks. The usual maintenance dosage is 100 to 150 mg/day in 2 divided doses.

The differences in doses are caused by metabolic drug interactions (see following). The slow initiation of therapy is to reduce risk of rash.

E. Formulations

Lamotrigine is available as scored tablets in the following strengths: 25, 100, 150, and 200 mg.

F. Toxicity

No unique side effects have been identified as presumably caused by lamotrigine. The following common side effects of antiepileptic drugs are increased in frequency or severity in some patients (especially those on carbamazepine) when lamotrigine is added: drowsiness, dizziness, diplopia, headache, ataxia, tremor, and nausea. Rash is an idiosyncratic toxicity occurring in 10% of patients, and progressing to Stevens–Johnson syndrome in some. The risk is 1/1,000 in most adults, 10/1,000 in adults taking valproic acid, and 10–20/1,000 in children. Long-term toxicity has not been reported.

G. Drug Interactions

Carbamazepine, phenytoin, phenobarbital, and primidone reduce the plasma concentration of lamotrigine. Lamotrigine does not affect the plasma concentration of carbamazepine, phenobarbital, phenytoin, primidone, or valproic acid. Valproic acid dramatically increases plasma concentration of lamotrigine.

When lamotrigine is added to carbamazepine, patients sometimes develop symptoms of carbamazepine toxicity (drowsiness, dizziness, diplopia). The plasma concentration of carbamazepine is unchanged, and there is disagreement as to whether the plasma concentration of carbamazepine epoxide (active metabolite) is elevated. This incompletely understood drug interaction is managed by reduction in carbamazepine dosing rate (often a reduction of 200 mg per day is adequate), and should not be mistaken for toxicity caused directly by recently added lamotrigine.

H. Pregnancy

There are no adequate studies of lamotrigine in pregnant women.

VII. PHENOBARBITAL

A. Mechanism of Action
See Section I and Table 11-1.

B. Indications, Advantages, and Disadvantages
Phenobarbital is FDA-approved as initial or adjunctive therapy for partial and tonic-clonic seizures. Parenteral phenobarbital is used for treatment of status epilepticus (see Chapter 12).

Serious toxicity is rare with phenobarbital. Parenteral administration is possible, and a loading dose may be given by the oral or intravenous route. Phenobarbital is inexpensive and need be taken only once a day by many adults. Phenobarbital is less effective than phenytoin or carbamazepine for partial seizures. Phenobarbital also causes sedation, irritability, hyperactivity (in children), and impairment of higher intellectual function in a higher percentage of patients.

The position of phenobarbital relative to other drugs approved for the same indications is reviewed in Chapter 10.

C. Pharmacokinetics (Table 11-1)
Phenobarbital is absorbed slowly (over 6 to 18 hr) but completely from the small intestine. The drug is 40% to 60% protein-bound. Approximately one-third of an administered dose of phenobarbital is excreted unchanged in the urine, and two-thirds is excreted as metabolites created by hepatic biotransformation. Phenobarbital exhibits linear (nonconcentration-dependent) pharmacokinetics with an elimination half-life of approximately 4 days in adults. Phenobarbital steady-state plasma concentration is attained 14 to 20 days after initiating therapy or changing dosing rate.

D. Usual Pediatric and Adult Dosages
See Tables 11-2 and 11-3.

E. Formulations
Phenobarbital is available as tablets (15, 30, 60, and 100 mg), elixir (20 mg/5 cc), and sodium phenobarbital for injection (65 mg/cc and 130 mg/cc).

F. Toxicity
Dose-related toxicity includes sedation, irritability, hyperactivity (in children), slowed mentation, and ataxia.

Rash is a common idiosyncratic toxicity, and agranulocytosis, aplastic anemia, and hepatitis are very rare idiosyncratic reactions. Long-term toxicity includes folic acid, vitamin K, and vitamin D deficiency.

G. Drug Interactions

The phenobarbital plasma concentration is increased after the addition of valproic acid. Phenobarbital may lower the plasma concentrations of carbamazepine, valproic acid, lamotrigine, bishydroxycoumarin, warfarin, theophylline, and cimetidine.

H. Disease States

The risk of phenobarbital intoxication must be monitored carefully in patients with renal or hepatic disease.

I. Pregnancy

Available reports are conflicting as to whether phenobarbital is or is not teratogenic when it is taken alone. Phenobarbital, in combination with other antiepileptic drugs, appears to increase the risk of teratogenesis.

VIII. PHENYTOIN (DILANTIN)

A. Mechanism of Action

See Section I and Table 11-1.

B. Indications, Advantages, and Disadvantages

Phenytoin is indicated for initial or adjunctive treatment of complex partial or tonic-clonic seizures. Phenytoin was found to be one of the two safest and most effective drugs for these seizure types in comparative studies of older drugs (carbamazepine is the other). Phenytoin also is effective for generalized-onset tonic-clonic seizures. Parenteral phenytoin is used for treatment of status epilepticus (see Chapter 12). Phenytoin is relatively nonsedating (sedation is mild and similar to that of carbamazepine), and serious toxicity is rare. Parenteral administration of phenytoin is possible, and a loading dose may be given by the oral, intramuscular, or intravenous route. Phenytoin need be taken only once a day by many adults and is inexpensive. Use of phenytoin may result in reversible gingival hyperplasia and other cosmetic side effects (hirsutism, acne, coarsening of facial features; not conclusively proven to be caused by phenytoin).

C. Pharmacokinetics (See Table 11-1)

Approximately 85% of an orally administered dose of brand-name phenytoin (Dilantin 100-mg extended-release Kapseals) is absorbed slowly over a period of 24 hours. Intramuscular sodium phenytoin for injection is slowly and erratically absorbed; while the fosphenytoin preparation (see below) is rapidly and completely absorbed by the intramuscular route. Phenytoin is 69% to 96% protein bound and is biotransformed by the liver. Phenytoin has concentration-dependent (nonlinear) pharmacokinetics that have the following consequences: (a) plasma concentration increases (or decreases) faster than the dosing rate when the dosing rate is increased (or decreased); (b) the time to reach steady state after a change in the dosing rate may vary from 5 to 28 days; and (c) the plasma concentration at one dosing rate does not directly predict the plasma concentration at another dosing rate.

D. Formulations

1. Oral

Phenytoin is available in 30- and 100-mg capsules and 50-mg tablets. Note that the only extended-release form of phenytoin (approved for once daily administration) is the brand-name Dilantin, 100 mg Kapseals. A syrup for oral dosage (125 mg/5 cc) is available.

2. Parenteral

Parenteral preparations include injectable sodium phenytoin (injectable Dilantin and generic) (50 mg/cc) and fosphenytoin (Cerebyx) (50 mg phenytoin equivalent/cc).

Standard injectable sodium phenytoin is poorly soluble in water. When injected into muscle, it is slowly and unpredictably absorbed and may cause local tissue damage. Fosphenytoin is a water-soluble phosphate ester of phenytoin that is rapidly and predictably absorbed by the intramuscular route and causes minimal local tissue damage. Thus, fosphenytoin is preferable to injectable sodium phenytoin for intramuscular administration. Once in the circulation, fosphenytoin is cleaved by alkaline phosphatase in red blood cells and liver to yield phenytoin. Fosphenytoin by the intramuscular route may be used in place of oral or intravenous phenytoin for short-term maintenance dosing or for administration of a loading dose.

Phenytoin may be administered by the intravenous route for maintenance dosing or for administration of a loading dose. Standard, injectable sodium phenytoin is insoluble in standard intravenous fluids (requiring undiluted direct administration) and may cause local irritation and phlebitis at the infusion site. Fosphenytoin is the preferred preparation because it is freely soluble in all standard intravenous fluids and causes less local irritation.

Parenteral phenytoin, fosphenytoin, and loading-dose procedures are discussed in detail in Chapter 12.

E. Usual Pediatric and Adult Dosages (See Tables 11-2 and 11-3)

The usual adult starting dose of phenytoin is 300 mg once daily, using an extended-release formulation (Dilantin Kapseals). The following persons should receive Dilantin Kapseals in two divided doses daily: (a) persons who have unacceptable toxicity associated with peak plasma concentration with once daily administration; (b) children (children have shorter phenytoin elimination half-lives than adults); and (c) persons not obtaining complete seizure control with once-daily administration (seizures may occur at the time of trough-plasma concentration). Persons receiving a prompt-release phenytoin preparation (i.e., a preparation that is not an extended-release preparation, all current, generic phenytoin products) should use a twice-daily regimen. Because of phenytoin's concentration-dependent pharmacokinetics, the authors use two special rules for titrating dosage: (a) daily dosing rates should be changed by only 30 or 50 mg when the phenytoin-plasma concentration is 10 µg per ml or higher; (b) one should wait 28 days for attainment of steady-state plasma concentration after a change in dosing rate.

F. Toxicity

Local toxicity includes gastric distress (can often be alleviated by taking medication with meals).

Common dose-related side effects are nystagmus, ataxia, dysarthria, and sedation. High plasma concentration may be associated with changes in mental state ranging from dysphoria and mild confusion to coma, choreiform movements, and increased seizure frequency. Idiosyncratic toxicity commonly includes rash (usually morbilliform and appearing within the first 12 weeks of therapy). Rare side effects include: agranulocytosis, thrombocytopenia, aplastic anemia, Stevens-Johnson syndrome, hepatitis, nephritis, lymphoma-like syndrome, thyroiditis, SLE, and hyperglycemia. Gingival hyperplasia occurs in approximately 20% of patients taking long-term phenytoin. The gingival hyperplasia can be treated with good oral hygiene or, rarely, gingivectomy. The gingival hyperplasia usually resolves within a few months if phenytoin is discontinued. Hirsutism, acne, and coarsening of facial features have all been attributed to phenytoin, but definitive scientific evidence for a cause-and-effect relationship with phenytoin has never been published for any of these. The following laboratory abnormalities (usually asymptomatic) have been associated with long-term phenytoin administration: decreased levels of folic acid, vitamin K, vitamin D, and immunoglobulin A; decreased bone density; decreased motor nerve conduction velocity; and increased plasma-alkaline phosphatase levels.

G. Drug Interactions

Adding phenytoin may increase the plasma concentration of warfarin with a resulting increase in prothrombin time. Adding phenytoin may decrease the plasma concentrations of carbamazepine, valproic acid, felbamate, lamotrigine, methadone, theophylline, bishydroxycoumarin, and oral contraceptives. The following drugs may raise the plasma concentration of phenytoin: carbamazepine, felbamate, cimetidine, bishydroxy coumarin, chloramphenicol, isoniazid and disulfiram. The following drugs may lower the plasma concentration of phenytoin: rifampin, antacids and valproic acid (free-phenytoin plasma concentration is unchanged).

H. Disease States

Phenytoin intoxication is not likely in patients with renal disease, but relatively high plasma concentrations of unbound drug are present and may need to be specifically determined at times. There is some risk of phenytoin intoxication in hepatic dysfunction.

I. Pregnancy

In common with several other antiepileptic drugs, there is a 2% to 3% increased risk of fetal epilepsy syndrome in infants born to mothers taking phenytoin.

IX. PRIMIDONE (MYSOLINE)

A. Mechanism of Action
See Section I and Table 11-1.

B. Indications, Advantages, and Disadvantages
Primidone is indicated for use as initial or adjunctive therapy of simple partial, complex partial, or tonic-clonic seizures. Serious toxicity is rare with primidone. Primidone is less effective than phenytoin or carbamazepine for these types of seizures. A high incidence of toxicity is seen at the time of initiation of therapy (nausea, dizziness, ataxia, somnolence). Primidone causes disabling sedation, irritability, and/or impairment of high intellectual function during chronic administration in a relatively high percentage of patients. Parenteral administration of primidone is not possible, and a loading dose cannot be administered by the oral or intravenous route. The drug is administered in a thrice-daily regimen.

C. Pharmacokinetics (Table 11-1)
Primidone is rapidly absorbed from the gastrointestinal tract. Protein binding is minimal. Biotransformation of primidone leads to the formation of two metabolites, phenobarbital and phenylethymalonamide. Each has antiepileptic activity along with primidone per se. The rate of conversion to phenobarbital is enhanced by concurrent use of enzyme-inducing drugs, such as phenytoin. When primidone is given as monotherapy, the derived phenobarbital concentration may be less than the serum concentration of primidone. Concurrent use of inducing drugs often produces plasma concentrations of primidone that are one-third those of the metabolically derived phenobarbital. Concurrent use of primidone and phenobarbital should be avoided to prevent phenobarbital toxicity (this is further enhanced if a third drug with metabolic induction qualities is used).

D. Usual Pediatric and Adult Dosages (See Tables 11-2 and 11-3)
Special care is needed with the initiation of therapy. Patients need to be forewarned about side effects such as dizziness, nausea, sedation, and ataxia. Patients 8 years of age and older may be started according to the following schedule: days 1 to 3, 100 to 150 mg at bedtime; days 4 to 6, 100 to 125 mg b.i.d.; days 7 to 9, 100 to 125 mg t.i.d.; day

10, 250 mg t.i.d. A t.i.d. regimen usually is used to reduce side effects associated with peak-plasma concentrations.

E. Formulations
Fifty and 250 mg tablets and a suspension (250 mg/5 cc) are available.

F. Toxicity
Common side effects are: dysphoria, sedation, dizziness, and ataxia, especially when initiating therapy. Idiosyncratic toxicity includes rash and, very rarely, leukopenia and thrombocytopenia, agranulocytosis and aplastic anemia, lymphadenopathy, hepatitis, and SLE. Prolonged therapy may be associated with folic acid, vitamin D, and vitamin K deficiency.

G. Drug Interactions
Valproic acid and isoniazid may increase the plasma concentrations of primidone. Carbamazepine and phenytoin increase the plasma concentration of the phenobarbital-derived from primidone. Primidone decreases the plasma concentration of carbamazepine, lamotrigine, and valproic acid.

H. Disease States
The risk of primidone toxicity is enhanced in instances of renal disease. Its effect in patients with hepatic disease is less clear.

X. TOPIRAMATE (TOPAMAX)
A. Mechanisms of Action
See Section I and Table 11-1.

B. Indications, Advantages, and Disadvantages
Topiramate is indicated as adjunctive therapy for partial seizures in adults which are not controlled with first-choice drugs, such as carbamazepine or phenytoin. The six drugs used for this indication are compared in Table 10-2. Topiramate had the highest reported responder rate in controlled trials for refractory partial seizures. Topiramate has few drug interactions and may be given twice per day.

Central nervous system side effects are not uncommon with topiramate. Renal stones occurred in 1.5% of study patients. Topiramate is more expensive than older drugs.

C. Pharmacokinetics (see Table 11-1)

Topiramate is rapidly absorbed with peak-plasma concentrations occurring 1 to 4 hours after oral administration. Oral bioavailability is greater than 80% and unaffected by food or dosage size. Protein binding is approximately 15%. In the absence of enzyme-inducing drugs, 80% of a dose is excreted unchanged in the urine with an elimination half-life of 20 to 30 hr. In the presence of enzyme-inducing drugs, 50% to 80% of a dose is excreted unchanged in the urine, with an elimination half-life of 12 to 15 hours. The metabolic products of topiramate are formed in the liver and do not appear to be biologically active.

D. Usual Adult Dosage

The recommended total dose as adjunctive therapy is 400 mg/day in two divided doses. A daily dosage of 200 mg/day has inconsistent effects and is less effective than 400 mg/day. It is recommended that therapy be initiated at 50 mg/day, followed by titration to an effective dose. Daily dosages above 1,600 mg have not been studied. At the time of publication of this book topiramate did not have an approved indication for use in children.

E. Formulations

Twenty-five, 100, and 200 mg tablets are available.

F. Toxicity

The most common side effects with topiramate are CNS related: drowsiness, dizziness, decreased attention or impaired concentration, paresthesia, nervousness, confusion and impaired memory. These side effects usually are mild to moderate, develop during the first weeks of therapy and may decline over time. Minor weight loss occurs in some patients.

Renal stones occurred in 1.5% of study patients. Renal-stone risk does not appear to be related to duration or dosage of therapy, and may be related to individual patient susceptibility. A previous history or family history or stones may be a contraindication to topiramate.

Hepatotoxicity and bone-marrow depression have not been observed. It is not necessary to monitor tests of liver or bone marrow function.

G. Drug Interactions

Enzyme-inducing drugs (phenytoin, carbamazepine, phenobarbital) significantly reduce topiramate blood levels. Valproic acid has no effect upon topiramate blood levels. Topiramate may increase phenytoin blood levels, but has no effects on carbamazepine or phenytoin blood levels.

H. Disease States

Topiramate dosing rate may need to be reduced in patients with renal impairment or hepatic impairment. Topiramate is cleared rapidly by hemodialysis; a supplemental dose of topiramate may be required during hemodialysis.

I. Pregnancy

There are no adequate studies of topiramate in pregnant women.

XI. VALPROIC ACID (DEPAKENE, DEPAKOTE)

A. Mechanism of Action

See Section I and Table 11-1.

B. Indications, Advantages, and Disadvantages

Valproic acid is FDA-approved as initial or adjunctive therapy of absence seizures and for adjunctive use in patients with multiple seizure types (usually tonic-clonic and/or myoclonic) which include absence seizures. Valproic acid also is FDA-approved as monotherapy or adjunctive therapy for the treatment of complex partial seizures occuring alone, or in association with other seizure types. The role of valproic acid in treating absence seizures and partial seizures is reviewed in Chapter 10.

C. Pharmacokinetics (see Table 11-1)

Valproic acid is rapidly and completely absorbed after oral administration, with a slight delay in absorption if taken after meals. The drug is approximately 90% protein-bound. Protein binding varies with drug plasma concentration, and the free fraction increases with increasing plasma concentration. Primary metabolism is by hepatic hydroxylation and conjugation with glucuronide. Valproic acid also appears in the bowel and undergoes enterohepatic circulation. Beta- and omega-oxidation may also take place. Excretion as glucuronide in the urine follows, with minor amounts lost in feces and expired air.

D. Usual Pediatric and Adult Dosages (See Tables 11-2 and 11-3)

The package insert recommends starting at 15 mg kg per day, but many experts start at a lower dosing rate to reduce start-up toxicity. Dosage is gradually increased by 5 to 10 mg/per kg per day every week until therapeutic success is achieved, until a maximum dose of 60 mg per kg per day is reached, or until the plasma concentration exceeds 150 µg per ml.

E. Formulations

Valproic acid (Depakene and generics) is available in 250 mg capsules and as a syrup (250 mg/5 cc). It is also available as enteric-coated divalproex sodium, a stable coordinate compound (Depakote), in 125, 250, and 500 tablets and a sprinkle form which can be mixed with food. Valproic acid must be administered in three or more divided doses per day. Divalproex sodium can usually be administered twice daily and produces fewer gastrointestinal side effects than valproic acid in many patients, but is more expensive.

An intravenous preparation (Depacon) is available for patients for whom drug administration is temporarily not possible. Depacon contains the equivalent of 100 mg valproic acid per milliliter, must be diluted, must be infused slowly, and must be given in divided doses (see package insert for details).

F. Toxicity

Local toxicity includes anorexia, nausea, and indigestion. These symptoms may be reduced with the divalproex sodium preparations. Dose-related toxicities are action tremor (40% of adults, less frequent in children), elevated plasma transaminase (usually transient but may be a harbinger of serious hepatic disease), and hyperammonemia. Idiosyncratic toxicity includes hepatic necrosis, thrombocytopenia, pancreatitis (0.5%), stupor and coma, so-called "worsened" behaviors, and depression. The risk of hepatic fatality is greatest in children younger than 11 years of age and in persons taking valproic acid in combination with other antiepileptic drugs. Long-term toxicities are weight gain (20%), hair loss (4%), and platelet dysfunction.

G. Drug Interactions

Valproic acid raises the plasma concentration of lamotrigine and phenobarbital. Phenytoin, phenobarbital, and carbamazepine lower the plasma concentration of valproic acid. Felbamate increases the plasma concentration of valproic acid.

H. Disease States

The use of valproic acid is best avoided in the presence of liver disease. Because of possible effects of valproic acid on hemostasis (thrombocytopenia, platelet dysfunction), persons taking valproic acid who are about to undergo surgery should have a through hemostasis evaluation.

I. Pregnancy

In common with several other antiepileptic drugs, valproic acid may increase the risk of fetal epilepsy syndrome. In addition, there is 2% risk of spina bifida in infants born to mothers taking valproic acid (vs 1 in 1,500 in the normal population).

XII. VIGABATRIN (SABRIL)

Vigabatrin was not approved by the FDA at the time this book was written, but may be approved shortly after this book is published. Information in this chapter is preliminary. The reader is referred to the package insert for the drug after the drug is approved for final information, especially on indications, warnings, and dosing.

A. Mechanism of Action

Vigabatrin is an irreversible inhibitor of GABA-transaminase, the only enzyme which breaks down GABA in the human brain. This results in increased concentration of the inhibitory neurotransmitter GABA in the brain.

B. Indications, Advantages, and Disadvantages

The first indication for which FDA approval is being sought is as adjunctive therapy for partial seizures. Vigabatrin has proven effective in several controlled trials for this indication. Vigabatrin has no serious hypersensitivity side effects, has few drug interactions, and may be given once or twice per day. Vigabatrin has fairly common neurologic side effects (drowsiness, dizziness, ataxia, headaches) and may precipitate a severe reversible psychosis in a small percentage of patients.

C. Pharmacokinetics

Vigabatrin is a racemic drug, and only the s-enantiomer is biologically active. Maximum plasma concentrations are reached 0.5 to 3 hr after oral administration. Oral bioavailability is greater than 65% and not effected by food. Vigabatrin crosses the blood–brain barrier. The drug is eliminated unchanged by the kidneys with an elimination half-life of approximately 7 hr. The duration of biologic activity depends upon the rate of synthesis of new GABA-transaminase. Clinical experience indicates the effects of vigabatrin reverse 1 to 4 days after the drug is discontinued. There is no established therapeutic range for vigabatrin-plasma concentration.

D. Usual Adult Dosage
In clinical trials, the usual starting dose was 1 gm per day (q.d. or b.i.d. schedule). If necessary, the daily dosage was increased in 0.5 or 1.0 gm increments at weekly intervals, depending upon clinical response and tolerability. A daily dosage of 3.0 gm produced good results in many studies. Maximum daily dosage was usually 4 to 6 gm per day.

E. Toxicity
Drowsiness and fatigue are the most common side effects of vigabatrin (20% incidence). Less common (>5% incidence) CNS-side effects include: dizziness, headache, diplopia, ataxia, vertigo, confusion, and insomnia. Psychiatric side effects include nervousness, depression, aggression, hyperactivity, and agitation. Severe behavioral disturbances, including psychosis and encephalopathy, have developed in some patients. Approximately 5% of patients discontinue vigabatrin because of psychiatric side effects. Abrupt withdrawal of vigabatrin has resulted in withdrawal seizures, agitation, hallucinations, and delusional thinking. Weight gain, abdominal pain, nausea, and constipation have been reported.

F. Drug Interactions
Phenytoin plasma concentration may decrease when vigabatrin is added. Otherwise, vigabatrin has few drug interactions.

G. Disease States
Vigabatrin dosing rate may need to be reduced in patients with renal impairment.

H. Pregnancy
There are no adequate studies of vigabatrin in pregnant women.

XIII. LESS COMMONLY USED ANTIEPILEPTIC DRUGS

The following drugs are occasionally used in treating partial (localization-related) and tonic-clonic seizures: acetazolamide (Diamox), chlorazepate (Tranxene), diazepam (Valium), ethotoin (Peganone), felbamate (Felbatol), mephenytoin (Mesantoin), mephobarbital (Mebaral), and phenacemide (Phenurone). The following drugs are occasionally used in treating absence seizures: acetazolamide (Diamox), diazepam (Valium), methsuximide (Celontin), paramethadione (Paradione), phensuximide (Milontin), trimethadione (Tridione). In general, the less commonly used drugs are less safe, less effective, or less convenient than commonly used drugs. The less commonly used drugs are usually prescribed by persons with expertise in epilepsy and are described in more detail in references cited at the end of this chapter [Browne (4) and Levy et al. (12)].

XIV. GENERIC ANTIEPILEPTIC DRUGS

The American Academy of Neurology has reviewed the topic of generic antiepileptic drugs. They recommend that for two drugs, carbamazepine and phenytoin, patients should remain on the same preparation made by the same manufacturer because of theoretical and documented risks of therapeutic inequivalence when switching among different manufacturers' preparations. For the other antiepileptic drugs, there are no generic preparations or the generic preparations appear to be performing adequately.

XV. OTHER EXPERIMENTAL ANTIEPILEPTIC DRUGS

Clobazam, levetiracetam (ucb L-059), oxcarbamazepine, tiagabine, and zonisamide are experimental drugs for epilepsy at the time this chapter is being written. See reviews of Dichter and Brodie (8) and Fisher and Blum (11) for details.

REFERENCES

1. Binnie CD. Lamotrigine. In: Engel J, Pedley TA, eds. *Epilepsy: a comprehensive textbook*. Philadelphia: Lippincott–Raven, 1997.
2. Brodie MJ, Dichter MA. Established antiepileptic drugs. *N Engl J Med* 1996;334:168–175.
3. Browne TR. Phenytoin and other hydantoins. In: Engel J, Pedley TA, eds. *Epilepsy: a comprehensive textbook*. Philadelphia: Lippincott–Raven, 1997.

4. Browne TR. Less commonly used antiepileptic drugs. In: Engel J, Pedley TA, eds. *Epilepsy: a comprehensive textbook*. Philadelphia: Lippincott–Raven, 1997.
5. Browne TR. Fosphenytoin. *Clin Neuropharmacol* 1997;20:1–4.
6. Chadwick DW. New options for the treatment of epilepsy: topiramate in perspective. *Epilepsia* 1997; 38(suppl 1):S1–S62.
7. Chadwick D, Browne TR. Gabapentin. In: Engel J, Pedley TA, eds. *Epilepsy: a comprehensive textbook*. Philadelphia: Lippincott–Raven, 1997.
8. Dichter MA, Brodie MJ. New antiepileptic drugs. *N Engl J Med* 1996;334:1583–1590.
9. Engel J, Pedley TA, eds. *Epilepsy: a comprehensive textbook*. Philadelphia: Lippincott–Raven, 1997, Chapters 128–158.
10. Faught E, Wilder BJ, Ramsay RE, et al. Topiramate placebo-controlled dose-ranging trial in refractory partial epilepy using 200-, 400- and 600-mg daily dosages. *Neurology* 1996;46:1684–1690.
11. Fisher R, Blum D. Clobazam, tiagabine, topiramate, and other new antiepileptic drugs. *Epilepsia* 1995; 36(suppl 2):S105–S114.
12. Levy RH, Mattson RH, Meldrum BS, eds. *Antiepileptic drugs*, 4th ed. New York: Raven Press, 1995.
13. Macdonald RL, Meldrum B. Principles of antiepileptic drug action. In: Levy RH, Mattson RH, Meldrum BS, eds. *Antiepileptic drugs*, 4th ed. New York: Raven Press, 1995.
14. MacKenzie RA, ed. The use of vigabatrin in epilepsy. *Neurology* 1996;47(Suppl 1):1–16.
15. Mattson RH. Carbamazepine. In: Engel J, Pedley TA, eds. *Epilepsy: a comprehensive textbook*. Philadelphia: Lippincott–Raven, 1997.
16. Mattson RH and the Department of Veterans Affairs Epilepsy Cooperative Study #118 Group. A comparison of carbamazepine, phenobarbital, phenytoin and primidone in partial and secondarily generalized tonic-clonic seizures. *N Engl J Med* 1985;313: 145–151.
17. Mattson RH and the Department of Veterans Affairs Epilepsy Cooperative Study No. 264 Group. A comparison of valproate with carbamazepine for the treatment of complex partial seizures and secondarily generalized tonic-clonic seizures in adults. *N Engl J Med* 1992;327:765–771.

18. Nuwer M, Browne TR, Dodson WE, et al. American Academy of Neurology Position Statement: generic substitution for antiepileptic medication. *Neurology* 1990;40:1641–1643.
19. Sommerville K. Tiagabine. In: Engel J, Pedley TA, eds. *Epilepsy: a comprehensive textbook.* Philadelphia: Lippincott–Raven, 1997.
20. Wyllie E, ed. *The treatment of epilepsy: principles and practices,* 2nd ed. Baltimore: Williams and Wilkins, 1997, Chapters 49–73.

STATUS EPILEPTICUS

I. OVERVIEW

A. Definitions

Status epilepticus is defined as a condition in which seizures occur so frequently that the patient does not fully recover from one seizure before having another. Status epilepticus is also defined as a single seizure lasting 30 min or longer. There are several types of status epilepticus, depending upon seizure type: tonic-clonic (grand mal), simple partial (focal), complex partial (psychomotor, temporal lobe), and absence (petit mal). Tonic-clonic status epilepticus is the most common and most life-threatening type of status epilepticus.

B. Epidemiology

The frequency of status epilepticus occurrences (all types) is 50 per 100,000 population per year or 125,000 occurrences per year in the United States. Frequency is highest in children and in adults older than 60 years. In both children and adults approximately 80% of cases are of the tonic-clonic type. Approximately one-third of cases fall into each of three groups: (a) first unprovoked seizure, (b) patients with well-established epilepsy, (c) acute new neurologic disease. The life-time incidence of status epilepticus among patients with known seizure disorders is 1% to 4%, and is highest in patients with localization-related/symptomatic (partial, focal) epilepsy.

II. TONIC-CLONIC STATUS EPILEPTICUS

A. Clinical Presentation

Tonic-clonic status epilepticus generally follows a predictable sequence of events (Fig. 12-1) which can be described in three categories: motor, electroencephalographic (EEG), and systemic. In both human and animal studies, the phenomenology of these phases differs between early tonic-clonic status epilepticus (Phase I) and late tonic-clonic status epilepticus (Phase II). The transition from Phase I to Phase II usually occurs after 30 to 60 min.

1. Motor Events, Phase I

These consist of a tonic phase (muscles continuously contracted) followed by a clonic phase (alternate contrac-

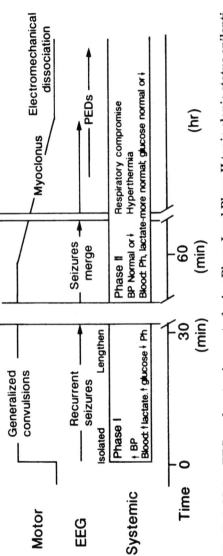

Fig. 12-1. Motor, EEG, and systemic events during Phase I and Phase II tonic-clonic status epilepticus. From Ref. 3 with permission.

tion and relaxation of muscles). The seizures are bilaterally synchronous at onset in 45% of patients; in the remainder they are aversive (head and/or eyes turned to one side) or focal at onset.

2. Motor Events, Phase II

As tonic-clonic status epilepticus continues, seizures often become shorter in duration and more restricted in distribution. Focal or lateralized motor activity may occur and does not necessarily imply focal pathology. Later the motor activity may be reduced to brief muscle jerks (myoclonus). Finally, there may be no motor activity occurring at times when prominent paroxysmal activity is present on the EEG (electromechanical dissociation).

3. EEG Events

A progressive succession of five EEG patterns occurs in patients with tonic-clonic status epilepticus: (a) discrete clinical and EEG seizures with interictal slowing; (b) waxing and waning of ictal discharges; (c) continuous ictal discharge; (d) continuous ictal discharges punctuated by flat periods; and (e) periodic epileptiform discharges (PEDs) on a flat background. In later stages electromechanical dissociation may be present.

4. Systemic Events

The principal systemic events occurring during tonic-clonic status epilepticus are summarized in Figure 12-1. Additional events may include: oral trauma, head trauma, aspiration pneumonia, orthopedic injuries (especially compression fractures of thoracic or lumbar vertebrae), myoglobinuria (caused by muscle breakdown during seizures), pulmonary edema, cardiac arrhythmias, myocardial infarction, dehydration, disseminated intravascular coagulation, leucocytosis, and cerebrospinal fluid (CSF) pleocytosis. These last two events, combined with fever, may spuriously suggest a central nervous system (CNS) infection.

5. Clinical Significance of Phase II Tonic-Clonic Status Epilepticus

Phase II status epilepticus has four clinically significant aspects. First, the initial presentation (to the treating physician) of tonic-clonic status epilepticus can be a comatose patient with or without myoclonic jerks if the patients has had preceding tonic-clonic seizures, or has had only a few tonic-clonic seizures after a severe cerebral insult. Second, brain damage during experimental models of tonic-clonic status epilepticus occurs only during Phase

II, and not during Phase I. Third, Phase II tonic-clonic epilepticus is more difficult to control with drugs than Phase I. Fourth, these observations argue for aggressive therapy during Phase I of tonic-clonic status epilepticus.

B. Pathophysiology

Several factors appear to account for the prolongation of the epileptic state in tonic-clonic and partial status epilepticus: (a) changes in extracellular environment (e.g., increased potassium); (b) increase in excitatory AMPA (alpha-amino-3-hydroxy-5-methyl-4-isoxazolepropionic acid) and NMDA (N-methyl-D-aspartate) neurotransmission; (c) decrease in inhibitory GABA (gamma-aminobutyric acid) neurotransmission; (d) activation of voltage-gated calcium channels. See Fountain and Lothman (6) for more detailed review.

C. Prognosis

1. Mortality

The mortalities of status epilepticus in the pediatric, adult, and elderly populations are 2.5%, 14%, and 38%, with an overall rate of 22%. Death may be caused by the basic disease process causing status epilepticus, medical complications, or overmedication. The mortality related to prolonged seizures per se is 2% to 5%.

2. Brain Damage and Cerebral Dysfunction

There is a large amount of animal literature demonstrating that prolonged tonic-clonic or partial seizures may result in permanent brain damage through multiple mechanisms. Permanent damage does not occur following Phase I tonic-clonic status epilepticus, but does occur following Phase II tonic-clonic status epilepticus in animals. However, there are virtually no studies that systematically evaluate neurologic outcome after status epilepticus in an unselected human population. Less than definitive reports suggest tonic-clonic or partial status epilepticus may sometimes be accompanied by permanent neurologic and/or cognitive sequelae in humans. On the basis of these considerations, it is generally assumed that prolonged tonic-clonic or complex partial seizures may cause brain damage or cognitive dysfunction in humans, and should be prevented with vigorous therapy. The reviews of Browne et al. (3) and De Lorenzo et al. (4) cited at the end of this chapter cover this topic in more detail.

D. Treatment of Tonic-Clonic Status Epilepticus

The treatment plan below is based upon the plan of the Working Group on Status Epilepticus of the Epilepsy Foundation of America published in 1993 and is summarized in Table 12-1. The only modifications are inclusion of fosphenytoin and results from a Veterans Administration Cooperative Study (12), which were not available when the plan was formulated.

1. Immediate Treatment

As with any unresponsive patient, initial management of status epilepticus includes the ABCs of life support (maintaining an airway, supporting breathing, maintaining circulation), gaining access to circulation, and when possible, identifying and treating the probable cause. Body temperature, blood pressure, the electrocardiogram (ECG), and respiratory function should be monitored closely as soon as status epilepticus is recognized. Status epilepticus should be managed in an emergency department or in an environment in which continuous skilled nursing care is available.

A. AIRWAY AND OXYGENATION. The head and mandible should be positioned to promote drainage of secretions, and if necessary, the airway should be suctioned to ensure patency. If feasible, without undue force, an oral airway should be inserted. Oxygen should be administered by nasal cannula or mask and bag-valve-mask ventilator. If the need for respiratory assistance persists after the patient has been ventilated by bag-valve-mask, endotracheal intubation should be considered. However, administering an antiepileptic drug is a top priority, because managing the airway and assisting respiration are much easier after the convulsion is stopped.

B. GLUCOSE. Although hypoglycemia is a rare cause of status epilepticus, it may complicate other predisposing conditions, such as alcoholism. In most cases of status epilepticus, several factors result in early hyperglycemia. This, in turn, promotes insulin secretion. Late in status epilepticus (usually after 2 hr) secondary hypoglycemia can occur. Consequently, all patients should have a prompt determination of blood glucose level. If hypoglycemia is documented or if it is impossible to obtain a measurement of blood glucose, intravenous (IV) glucose should be administered through an indwelling venous catheter. In adults, an initial bolus injection of 50 ml of 50% glucose is used. In children, 25% glucose, 2 ml/kg, is administered.

**TABLE 12-1. A Suggested Timetable
for the Treatment of Status Epilepticus**

Time (min)	Action
0–5	Diagnose status epilepticus by observing continued seizure activity or one additional seizure.
	Give oxygen by nasal cannula or mask; position patient's head for optimal airway patency; consider intubation if respiratory assistance is needed.
	Obtain and record vital signs at onset and periodically thereafter; control any abnormalities as necessary; initiate ECG monitoring.
	Establish an IV; draw venous blood samples for glucose level, serum chemistries, hematology studies, toxicology screens and determinations of antiepileptic drug levels.
	Assess oxygenation with oximetry or periodic arterial blood gas determinations.
6–9	If hypoglycemia is established or a blood glucose is unavailable, administer glucose; in adults, give 100 mg of thiamine first, followed by 50 ml of 50% glucose by direct push into the IV; in children, the dose of glucose is 2 ml/kg of 25% glucose.
10–60	Administer either 0.1 mg/kg of lorazepam at 2 mg/min (maximum dose of 8 mg) or 0.2 mg/kg of diazepam at 5 mg/min by IV; if diazepam is given, it can be repeated if seizures do not stop after 5 min.
	For all patients given diazepam and for patients who continue to seize after lorazepam, administer 15–20 mg/kg phenytoin equivalent of fosphenytoin no faster than 150 mg phenytoin equivalent/min in adults and 3 mg phenytoin equivalent/kg per min in children by IV; monitor ECG and blood pressure during the infusion. For patients who stop seizing after lorazepam administer 15–20 mg/kg phenytoin equivalent of fosphenytoin at a slower infusion rate (e.g., 50 mg phenytoin equivalent/min).
>60	If status does not stop after 20 mg/kg phenytoin equivalent of fosphenytoin, give additional doses of 5 mg phenytoin equivalent/kg to a maximum dose of 30 mg phenytoin equivalent/kg.
	If status persists, give 20 mg/kg of phenobarbital by IV at 100 mg/min; when phenobarbital is given after a benzodiazepine, the risk of apnea or hypopnea is great and assisted ventilation is usually required.
	If status persists, give anesthetic doses of drugs such as pentobarbital; ventilatory assistance and vasopressors are virtually always necessary.

Modified from ref. (10) with permission.

Intravenous thiamine, 100 mg, should precede glucose administration in adults.

C. BLOOD PRESSURE. During the first 30 to 45 min, status epilepticus usually produces hypertension; thereafter, blood pressure returns to normal or falls below baseline values. Systolic blood pressure should be maintained at normal or high-normal levels during prolonged status, using vasopressors if necessary.

D. IV FLUIDS. Overhydration should be avoided because it can exacerbate the cerebral edema usually present in tonic-clonic status epilepticus.

E. BLOOD WORK. Blood should be drawn for a complete blood cell count, serum chemistry studies (including glucose, sodium, calcium, magnesium and blood urea nitrogen determinations), and antiepileptic drug levels. Urine and blood samples should be obtained for toxicologic screening. Adequate oxygenation should be confirmed by oximetry or periodic arterial blood gas determinations. All patients in status epilepticus develop acidosis, but this usually resolves promptly when status terminates. Bicarbonate therapy is usually unnecessary, but should be considered when a patient has severe acidosis.

F. BODY TEMPERATURE. Increased body temperature—sometimes to a striking degree—occurs in many patients with status epilepticus, primarily as a result of increased motor activity. Rectal temperature should be monitored frequently throughout treatment.

G. IDENTIFY AND TREAT PRECIPITATING FACTORS. The majority of cases of tonic-clonic status epilepticus do not occur randomly or as a result of a massive new cerebral lesion. Rather, there is a specific precipitating factor that causes a patient with a known seizure disorder to develop status epilepticus at a specific time. The most frequent causes of tonic-clonic status epilepticus are withdrawal from antiepileptic drugs and fever. Other precipitating factors include: (a) withdrawal from alcohol or sedative drugs; (b) metabolic disorder (hypocalcemia, hyponatremia, hypoglycemia, hepatic or renal failure); (c) sleep deprivation; (d) acute new brain insult (meningitis, encephalitis, cerebrovascular accident, or trauma); and (e) drug intoxication (e.g., cocaine, amphetamines, phencyclidine, tricyclics, or isoniazid). The precipitating factors in a case of status epilepticus must always be vigorously sought and treated to facilitate seizure control and to be certain that any reversible cause of cerebral dysfunction is treated before it results in irreversible cerebral damage.

H. ROLE OF ELECTROCEPHALOGRAPHY. If available, EEG monitoring confirms the diagnosis of status epilepticus and the presence or absence of paroxysmal activity after treatment. This is useful information. Treatment should not be delayed because of EEG procedures, however, unless the EEG is needed to establish the diagnosis of status epilepticus.

2. *Pharmaceutical Treatment*

   A. PHARMACOLOGIC PRINCIPLES. The ideal therapeutic agent for status epilepticus should: (a) enter the brain rapidly; (b) have an immediate onset of antiepileptic action; (c) not significantly depress consciousness or respiratory function; (d) have a long duration of antiepileptic action so that seizures do not recur; and (e) effectively block the motor, cerebral (EEG), and systemic effects of status epilepticus. The rate of brain entry of a drug is directly proportional to nonprotein-bound drug plasma concentration, lipid solubility, and cerebral blood flow. Therefore, status epilepticus is treated by intravenous infusion (to obtain high plasma concentration) of lipid-soluble antiepileptic drugs.

   Drug volume of distribution increases with lipid solubility, and lipid-soluble drugs tend to redistribute out of the brain and plasma into body fat. To rapidly attain and then maintain a therapeutic plasma and brain concentration of drug, it is necessary to give a loading dose sufficient to attain the desired concentration throughout the volume of distribution.

   The loading dose of a drug can be computed using the simple equation:

$$\text{Loading dose (mg/kg)} = \frac{\text{desired concentration (mg/L)}}{\text{volume of distribution (L/kg)}}$$

   Thus, a dose of 20 mg/kg of phenytoin (volume of distribution 0.7 L/kg) will produce a plasma concentration of 28.6 mg/L (1 mg/L = 1 μg/ml). Equation 1 can also be used to determine the dose needed to elevate plasma concentration to a higher value by substituting the desired increase in plasma concentration for plasma concentration in equation 1. Thus, a dose of 5 mg/kg of phenytoin will elevate plasma concentration by 7 mg/L.

   B. AVAILABLE DRUGS. Diazepam, lorazepam, phenytoin, and phenobarbital are the four drugs commonly used to treat tonic-clonic status epilepticus (Table 12-2). Diazepam and lorazepam are the most lipid-soluble of the group, enter the brain most rapidly, and stop status epilepticus most rapidly. Therefore, diazepam or lorazepam usually are the first drugs administered to a patient in active status epilepticus. Phenytoin and phenobarbital have longer durations of action and are used for long-acting seizure control.

TABLE 12-2. The major drugs used to treat status epilepticus: intravenous (IV) doses, pharmacokinetics, and major toxicities*

	Diazepam	Lorazepam	Fosphenytoin[a] or phenytoin	Phenobarbital
Adult IV dose, mg/kg range [total dose]	0.15–0.25	0.1 [4–8 mg]	15–20	20
Pediatric IV dose, mg/kg range [total dose]	0.1–1.0	0.05–0.5 [1–4 mg]	20	20
Maximal administration rate, mg/min	5	2.0	150 fosphenytoin 50 phenytoin	100
Time to stop status, min	1–3	6–10	10–30	20–30
Effective duration of action, hr	0.25–0.5	>12–24	24	>48
Elimination half-life, hr	30	14	24	100
Volume of distribution, L/kg	1–2	0.7–1.0	0.5–0.8	0.7
Potential side effects				
Depression of consciousness	10–30 min	Several hours	None	Several days
Respiratory depression	Occasional	Occasional	Infrequent	Occasional
Hypotension	Infrequent	Infrequent	Occasional	Infrequent
Cardiac arrhythmias	—	—	In patients with heart disease	—

[a]Fosphenytoin doses are in phenytoin equivalent units.
Modified from ref. (10), with permission.

C. **BENZODIAZEPINES: DIAZEPAM AND LORAZEPAM.** Diazepam and lorazepam rapidly enter the brain and stop status epilepticus. This makes them initial drugs of choice in patients who are actively seizing. However, use of these agents in status epilepticus is associated with a 10% risk of cardiorespiratory depression. Therefore, in patients not actively seizing, benzodiazepines are omitted, and therapy is usually initiated with phenytoin or phenobarbital.

Diazepam is highly lipid-soluble and is rapidly taken up by fatty tissues. This results in a rapid drop of plasma and brain levels and recurrence of seizures within less than 1 hr. Therefore, administration of diazepam should be followed immediately by a loading dose of a long-lasting drug, usually phenytoin.

Lorazepam has a longer duration of action than diazepam (12 to 24 hr), but is not a long-term therapy for tonic-clonic seizures. In patients thought to be at risk for recurring tonic-clonic seizures (or patients whose status epilepticus is not controlled with lorazepam), a loading dose of IV phenytoin usually is given in addition to lorazepam. The longer duration of action of lorazepam (in comparison to diazepam) permits more time for completion of diagnostic studies and slow infusion of phenytoin.

Diazepam is FDA-approved for treatment of status epilepticus and lorazepam is not. Nevertheless, many experts prefer lorazepam because of its longer duration of action.

The pharmacokinetics, dosing, timing of administration, and side effects of diazepam and lorazepam are shown in Tables 12-1 and 12-2.

D. **PHENYTOIN AND FOSPHENYTOIN.** Phenytoin and phenobarbital are the only long-acting antiepileptic drugs for tonic-clonic and partial seizures which can be given as an IV loading dose. Phenytoin is the usual first-choice drug over phenobarbital in older children and adults because of less sedation after treatment of status epilepticus with phenytoin, and because phenytoin is preferred to phenobarbital for long-term treatment of seizures in this age group.

An IV loading dose of phenytoin can be administered using either of two preparations: injectable sodium phenytoin or fosphenytoin. Injectable sodium phenytoin is poorly water-soluble and is formulated in a vehicle containing concentrated sodium hydroxide (pH 11 to 12) and propylene glycol. This formulation is irritating to veins and does not dissolve in standard IV solutions. Intravenous sodium phenytoin should be injected undiluted into a large vein and flushed with normal saline to prevent phlebitis. Extravasated drug may cause local tissue damage.

Fosphenytoin is a phosphate-ester prodrug of phenytoin developed as a replacement for standard injectable sodium phenytoin. Fosphenytoin is a simple aqueous solution with a pH of 8.8. After absorption, phenytoin is cleaved from fosphenytoin by alkaline phosphatase in red blood cells and other tissues. Advantages of fosphenytoin are that: (1) it dissolves readily in any standard IV solution (allowing continuous infusion with less staff time and greater convenience); (2) fosphenytoin produces less local toxicity (pain, burning, itching) than injectable sodium phenytoin; and (3) fosphenytoin produces less hypotension with rapid IV infusion than injectable sodium phenytoin. For these reasons, fosphenytoin is now the preferred formulation. Fosphenytoin is labeled in "phenytoin equivalent" units. Such units describe the amount of phenytoin liberated from fosphenytoin. Injectable sodium phenytoin and fosphenytoin both deliver 50 mg of phenytoin per cc of solution, and fosphenytoin is labeled as "50 mg phenytoin equivalent per cc."

The loading dose of phenytoin is 20 mg/kg in adults; the reduced dose for elderly patients or patients with cardiac disease is 15 mg/kg. The maximum infusion rate in adults is 150 mg/min (phenytoin equivalent) of fosphenytoin or 50 mg/min of injectable sodium phenytoin, i.e., the maximum infusion rate is 3 times faster with fosphenytoin. Lesser rates should be used in children (Table 12-1).

Phenytoin may cause hypotension, especially in older patients with pre-existing cardiac disease or in severely ill patients with marginal baseline blood pressure. Phenytoin should be administered cautiously to patients with known cardiac conduction abnormalities. Human and animal work indicates that risk of hypotension varies directly with phenytoin-plasma concentration. Peak-plasma phenytoin concentration occurs approximately 30 min after initiating a loading dose with either sodium phenytoin for injection (infused at 50 mg/min), or fosphenytoin (infused at 150 mg/min phenytoin equivalent). Blood pressure should be monitored at least 30 min after administering a loading dose with either preparation. If significant hypotension develops, the infusion should be slowed or stopped. In any patient, the rate of administration should be slowed to reduce the risk of complications if seizures stop before the entire phenytoin dose is given. If feasible, the electrocardiogram should be observed during administration, and the rate of infusion should be slowed if the QT interval widens or if arrhythmias develop. Occasionally, phenytoin is associated with respiratory depression, although this is less common than with benzodiazepines or barbiturates. It is also less likely than sedative drugs to impair consciousness.

The pharmacokinetics, dosing, timing of administration, and side effects of phenytoin and fosphenytoin are shown in Tables 12-1 and 12-2.

Fosphenytoin and phenytoin are absorbed too slowly by the IM route for treatment of status epilepticus. However, it is possible to administer a loading dose of phenytoin using IM fosphenytoin for chronic administration. A loading dose of 9 to 12 mg/kg of IM fosphenytoin will produce a maximum phenytoin plasma concentration of 12 µg/ml in 4 hr.

E. PHENOBARBITAL. Phenobarbital is often used as the first-choice long-acting drug for tonic-clonic status epilepticus in children under 6 years of age because of a perception (unproven in controlled trials) that phenobarbital may be more effective than phenytoin in this age group. Phenobarbital is used in patients of all ages who fail to be controlled with phenytoin or who are allergic to phenytoin.

The recommended dosage of phenobarbital is 20 mg/kg, but additional increments may be necessary to stop the convulsions. If the convulsion subsides before the entire dose is given, the rate of administration can be slowed; but the full dose should be given to reduce the risk of seizure recurrence. Doses of this magnitude administered to patients without previous exposure to sedative drugs usually produce substantial sedation and, occasionally, apnea or hypopnea. Hypotension is a potential side effect of phenobarbital, especially if given in combination with benzodiazepine. Phenobarbital administration should be slowed if blood pressure begins to drop.

The pharmacokinetics, dosing, timing of administration, and side effects of phenobarbital are shown in Tables 12-1 and 12-2.

F. COMPARATIVE TRIALS OF DRUGS FOR TONIC-CLONIC STATUS EPILEPTICUS. Only two such trials have been performed. In the first trial [Leppik et al.(8)] patients received an unspecified loading dose of phenytoin. In addition patients were randomly assigned to receive either lorazepam (4 to 8 mg) or diazepam (10 to 20 mg). Results were similar for the diazepam and lorazepam groups: seizure control—83% vs 76% of patients; median latency of action—2 vs 3 min; respiratory distress, hypotension, sedation—12% vs 13% of patients.

The second trial [Treiman et al. (12)] compared phenytoin 18 mg/kg, diazepam 0.15 mg/kg followed by phenytoin 18 mg/kg, phenobarbital 15mg/kg, and lorazepam 0.1 mg/kg as initial therapy for Phase I and Phase II tonic-clonic status epilepticus. Success was defined as no clinical or electrical seizure activity from 20 to 60 min after the start of the intravenous infusion. Success rates for Phase I were similar for diazepam plus phenytoin (68%), phenobarbital (76%), and lorazepam (73%). Success rates were lower for phenytoin (40%). Success rates for Phase II were low for all drugs: diazepam plus phenytoin (11.1%), phenobarbital (28.0%), lorazepam (28.6%), phenytoin (0%). Long-term success rates were not reported.

These data do not completely establish the regimen of choice for tonic-clonic status epilepticus. However, the data do indicate lorazepam alone is effective for at least 60 min, and phenytoin alone does not stop seizures within 20 to 60 min in many patients. For active tonic-clonic status epilepticus, many experts now advocate a regimen of immediate administration of lorazepam followed by slow infusion of phenytoin if lorazepam is successful in stopping seizures, or rapid infusion of phenytoin if lorazepam is unsuccessful in stopping seizures.

G. REFRACTORY TONIC-CLONIC STATUS EPILEPTICUS. In general, a consultant neurologist should be called when the patient does not wake up, convulsions continue after the administration of a benzodiazepine and phenytoin, or diagnostic confusion exists during evaluation and treatment. EEG monitoring is also helpful under these conditions.

If status epilepticus does not respond to recommended initial doses of a benzodiazepine, phenytoin, and phenobarbital, consideration should be given to anesthetizing the patient to suppress the cerebral ictal discharge. This is usually achieved with a barbiturate such as pentobarbital [see Browne and Mikati (3) for details]. Additional doses of phenytoin greater than 30 mg/kg are contraindicated because high doses provoke seizure activity.

3. Diagnostic Studies

LUMBAR PUNCTURE. Central nervous system infection is a major consideration in any patient with fever and status, especially a young child. In most of these situations, a lumbar puncture (LP) should be performed unless a contraindication, such as severe intracranial hypertension, suspected cerebral mass lesion, or obstructed CSF flow (e.g., hydrocephalus), is present. Unless the suspicion of CNS infection is high, brain imaging (usually a computed tomographic [CT] scan) should be performed before an LP is performed in adults. Performing a CT scan before the LP is not a "must" recommendation; however, if meningitis is not suspected and the LP is done electively with other diagnoses in mind, the CT scan is recommended first. If meningitis is suspected but an LP cannot be performed expediently, antibiotics should be administered immediately, rather than delayed until an imaging test and LP can be arranged. Note that whereas approximately 20% of patients have CSF fluid pleocytosis with a white blood cell count of up to 80 x 10^6/L following status (so-called "benign postictal pleocytosis"), meningitis is rare in patients with status.

Although the presence of leukocytes in CSF samples usually does not indicate that the patient has a CNS infection, patients with CSF pleocytosis should be treated for suspected meningitis until the diagnosis is excluded by culture or other means.

4. Long-Term Antiepileptic Drug Therapy after Tonic-Clonic or Partial Status Epilepticus

Patients who were previously well-controlled on a tolerable regimen should be restarted on the same medications. If an episode of status epilepticus was caused by an identifiable precipitating factor (e.g., fever, drug withdrawal, drug interaction), the patient should be counseled in how to avoid the precipitating factor. If no precipitating factor was identified, higher doses of medication or new medications should be considered.

In patients with new seizures, or undertreated patients whose status epilepticus was controlled with phenytoin or phenytoin plus a benzodiazepine, continue phenytoin. The practice of switching patients (especially women and children) to carbamazepine or valproic acid does not seem justified because: (a) phenytoin and carbamazepine have equal efficacy for tonic-clonic and complex partial seizures in all published double-blind studies; (b) valproic acid has similar efficacy (or less) when compared with phenytoin for these indications and has greater toxicity; (c) phenytoin and carbamazepine have similar (modest) effects on cognition; (d) the risks of serious teratogenesis (especially spina bifida) now appear to be greater with carbamazepine and valproic acid; (e) gingival hyperplasia occurs in only approximately 20% of patients on phenytoin and is reversible; (f) the evidence that phenytoin (as opposed to epilepsy, genetics, and poor hygiene) causes other cosmetic side effects is weak when examined critically; and (g) switching between two effective drugs can result in a transient increase in seizure frequency.

Patients requiring both phenytoin and phenobarbital to control status epilepticus and who did not have an acute precipitating factor (e.g., fever, drug withdrawal) probably should be continued on this combination.

Persons not subject to spontaneous, recurring seizures (e.g., drug withdrawal, drug intoxication, intercurrent illness) should be tapered off antiepileptic drugs.

5. Brain Imaging

Most patients who have status should have brain imaging performed at some point. Whereas any adult who begins to have seizures should have brain imaging, not all children with seizures need to have imaging performed. In younger patients, the indications for imaging include seizures that begin after head trauma, partial (focal) seizures, focal neurologic signs, focal EEG abnormalities, or status epilepticus as the first manifestation of a seizure disorder. Most patients with established epilepsy that has already been thoroughly evaluated do not need another brain imaging procedure after a bout of status. Each patient should, however, be considered individually. Some patients with known epilepsy develop new problems, and brain imaging sometimes reveals a new cause for the seizures. Among the various imaging techniques, CT of the brain is the most widely available and can usually be obtained rapidly in an emergency. In most patients, CT scanning is sufficient. However, when the need for imaging is not urgent or when the patients has had previous imaging, magnetic resonance imaging is preferred because it provides more detailed images and occasionally reveals abnormalities that cannot be visualized on CT scans.

III. SIMPLE PARTIAL (FOCAL MOTOR) STATUS EPILEPTICUS

A. Clinical Presentation

Simple partial status epilepticus may occur in patients with chronic seizure disorders or as a presenting symptom of an acute neurologic event. Focal motor status epilepticus in patients with chronic seizure disorders tends to be localized to the face and eyes, or to the face and upper limbs. The facial seizures tend to be more clonic, whereas the seizures affecting the limbs are apt to be tonic-clonic. Even though the motor seizure activity remains localized, there may be some impairment of consciousness or autonomic disturbances.

B. Management

In managing focal motor status epilepticus, the relative risks and benefits of therapies must be weighted. Intravenous diazepam usually temporarily halts focal motor status epilepticus and an intravenous loading dose of fosphenytoin often completely ends the attack. However, there is some risk to administering intravenous diazepam or fosphenytoin, as mentioned earlier. If the focal motor seizures can be temporarily tolerated, it is less dangerous to administer an IM loading dose of fosphenytoin. Directions for using IV diazepam and IM and IV fosphenytoin are given in the preceding section on tonic-clonic status epilepticus.

IV. COMPLEX PARTIAL (PSYCHOMOTOR, TEMPORAL LOBE) STATUS EPILEPTICUS

A. Clinical Presentation

This form of status epilepticus may take two forms in patients of all ages: (a) a prolonged twilight state with partial responsiveness, impaired speech, and quasi-purposeful automatisms, or (b) a series of complex partial seizures with staring, total unresponsiveness, speech arrest, and stereotyped automatisms with a twilight state between seizures.

A third type of prolonged partial complex status epilepticus has been described in children. Symptoms have included repeated partial complex, simple partial and secondarily generalized seizures with intervening, at times prolonged, interictal periods of psychotic behavior, hallucinations, delusions, aphasia, and neurovegetative symptoms. Resistance or tachyphylaxis to antiepileptic medication is a prominent feature of this syndrome.

B. Management

Therapy of complex partial status epilepticus consists of administering an IV loading dose of fosphenytoin or phenobarbital. Intravenous diazepam (FDA-approved) or lorazepam (not FDA-approved) may rapidly end an attack but carry some risk. Intravenous diazepam or lorazepam is indicated when the ongoing complex partial seizure activity represents an immediate serious threat or makes it impossible to administer fosphenytoin or phenobarbital. Lorazepam is preferred by many experts because of its longer duration of action.

Animal studies indicate that nonconvulsive status epilepticus in animals can cause brain damage; and there is some evidence that prolonged complex partial epilepticus may result in permanent cognitive disability in humans. This type of status epilepticus should, therefore, be treated rapidly using a protocol similar to that described earlier for treatment of tonic-clonic status epilepticus.

V. ABSENCE (PETIT MAL) STATUS EPILEPTICUS

A. Clinical Presentation

The clinical presentation of absence status epilepticus is altered consciousness, often accompanied by mild clonic movements of the eyelids and hands, and automatisms of the face and hands. The alteration of consciousness may range from a vague feeling that can be recognized only subjectively to stupor. Attacks may last 30 min to 12 or more hours. Although absence seizures occur chiefly in children, a considerable percentage of cases of absence status epilepticus occurs in adults. Adults who have failed to "outgrow" absence seizures seem particularly prone toward developing absence status epilepticus, and some adults with previously undiagnosed absence seizures may present in absence status epilepticus without a history of a seizure disorder. The differential diagnosis of absence status epilepticus includes drug intoxication, psychosis, metabolic encephalopathy, structural brain lesion, late (Phase II) tonic-clonic status epilepticus, complex partial status epilepticus, and psychogenic seizures. The diagnosis of absence status epilepticus is definitively established with an EEG that shows spike-wave activity. The spike-wave activity may be continuous or discontinuous and may consist of regular 3 per second spike-wave or (more commonly) irregular 2 to 3 per second spike-wave and polyspike-wave activity.

B. Management

Intravenous diazepam (FDA-approved) or lorazepam (not FDA-approved) at doses shown in Table 12-2 will usually stop absence status epilepticus for a period of time. Lorezapam is preferred by many experts because of its longer duration of action. Therapy then continues with high dose oral treatment with an anti-absence medication (e.g., ethosuximide 250 mg q8h) and further intermittent doses of an IV benzodiazepine if needed.

REFERENCES

1. Browne TR. Fosphenytoin. *Clin Neuropharmacol* 1997;20:1–12.
2. Browne TR. The pharmacokinetics of agents used to treat status epilepticus. *Neurology* 1990;40(suppl 2): 28–31.
3. Browne TR, Mikati MA. Status epilepticus. In: Roper AH, ed. *Neurological and neurosurgical intensive care*, 3rd ed. New York: Raven Press, 1993.
4. DeLorenzo RJ, Pellock JM, Towne AR, et al. Epidemiology of status epilepticus. *J Clin Neurophysiol* 1995; 12:310–325.
5. Engel J, Pedley TA, eds. *Epilepsy: a comprehensive textbook*. Philadelphia: Lippincott–Raven, 1997, Chapters 55–66, 120.
6. Fountain NB, Lothman EW. Pathophysiology of status epilepticus. *J Clin Neurophysiol* 1995;25:326–342.
7. Gilliam FG. Status epilepticus. In: Wyllie E, ed. *The treatment of epilepsy: principles and practice*, 2nd ed. Baltimore: Williams and Wilkins, 1997.
8. Leppik IE, Derivan AT, Homan RW, et al. Double blind study of lorazepam and diazepam in status epilepticus. *JAMA* 1983;249:1452–1454.
9. Pellock JM. Status epilepticus. In: Dodson WE, Pellock JM, eds. *Pediatric Epilepsy*. New York: Demos, 1993.
10. Treatment of convulsive status epilepticus: recommendations of the Epilepsy Foundation of America's working group on status epilepticus. *JAMA* 1993;270: 854–859.
11. Treiman DM. Electroclinical features of status epilepticus. *J Clin Neurophysiol* 1995;12:343–362.
12. Treiman DM, Meyers PD, Walton NY, et al. Treatment of convulsive status epilepticus: a multicenter comparison of four drug regimens. Presented at 48th Annual Meeting of American Academy of Neurology, March 26, 1996.

SPECIAL CONSIDERATIONS: PREGNANCY, THE ELDERLY

I. PREGNANCY

A. Seizure Frequency

Epilepsy is the most frequently encountered neurologic disorder during pregnancy. Approximately one-fourth of women with epilepsy will have an increase in seizure frequency during pregnancy. On occasion, some women will have seizures only during pregnancy. Seizure exacerbation may occur at any time, but is most frequently encountered at the end of the first and at the beginning of the second trimester. The likelihood of a change in seizure frequency appears to be independent of seizure type and frequency prior to pregnancy.

B. Pharmacologic Changes

While some women have an exacerbation of their seizures because of noncompliance or sleep deprivation, in the majority of women a number of physiological changes are responsible for the increase in seizure frequency. During pregnancy there is increased hepatic metabolism of most antiepileptic drugs, presumably because of a progesterone-stimulating effect on the liver. Body weight, total body water, and intravascular volume gradually increase through pregnancy. An increase in the volume into which the drug is distributed (volume of distribution) will result in a lower plasma concentration, even if the rate of drug metabolism or renal excretion is not altered. Lower plasma concentrations of antiepileptic drugs during pregnancy, therefore, appear to be related to the combined effect of enhanced hepatic metabolism and an increased volume of distribution.

Another important physiological change occurring during pregnancy is the change in protein binding of antiepileptic drugs. Plasma albumin concentration tends to decline during pregnancy which leads to a proportional reduction in the protein binding of drugs. Although the total plasma concentration of a drug may fall during pregnancy, the free (non-protein-bound) fraction of highly bound drugs such as phenytoin and valproate may increase, so that the concentration of free drug, which is the pharmacologically active portion, may change very little. To monitor effective drug concentration, it is sometimes necessary to measure concentrations of the free drug, especially for phenytoin and valproate.

C. Eclampsia

See Chapter 8.

D. Birth Defects and Teratogenesis of Antiepileptic Drugs

An association between fetal malformations, maternal epilepsy, and antiepileptic drugs has long been noted. In the late 1960s phenytoin was claimed to be associated with a number of birth anomalies, and the term "fetal hydantoin syndrome" was coined. However many of the birth anomalies associated with phenytoin were observed in infants of mothers with epilepsy who were on antiepileptic drugs other than phenytoin or who were not taking antiepileptic drugs. While antiepileptic drugs increase the risk for congenital anomalies, the risk of malformations is increased in mothers with epilepsy, regardless of whether they are taking antiepileptic drugs.

Major malformations include cleft lip and palate, cardiac defects (ventricular septal defects), neural tube defects, and urogenital defects. While congenital malformations in the general population range from 2% to 3%, the risk for malformations in infants of mothers with epilepsy is significantly higher. The risk if the mother is on antiepileptic drugs is even higher. The risk of malformations in any individual pregnancy in a women with epilepsy on a single antiepileptic drug, is estimated to be between 4% and 6% [Yerby and Collins (13)].

This risk of major malformations is also increased in mothers on polytherapy or toxic levels of antiepileptic drugs. All of the antiepileptic drugs have been associated with congenital malformations, although the incidence and type of the malformations may vary with the drug. Trimethadione, which should never be used during pregnancy, results in major malformations or fetal loss in 87% of pregnancies. This figure is far higher than for any other antiepileptic drugs. The risk of spina bifida appears to be significantly greater in infants exposed to valproate or carbamazepine but not other antiepileptic drugs.

In addition to major malformations, infants born to mothers on antiepileptic drugs are at increased risk for minor anomalies. These minor anomalies include epicanthal folds, hypertelorism, broad or flat nasal bridges, an upturned nasal tip, prominent lips, and fingernail hypoplasia. These minor anomalies, while more common than in the normal population, do not influence general health.

E. Other Complications of Pregnancy

Infants of mothers with epilepsy are approximately twice as likely to have an adverse pregnancy outcome. Stillbirths and neonatal death rates of infants of mothers with epilepsy are approximately twice as high as in the general population. Premature births are more common, and birth weights are also lower. Infants of mothers with epilepsy also have a higher risk of mental retardation, learning disabilities, and epilepsy than the normal population.

F. Breast Feeding

The concentration of a drug in breast milk is determined by the plasma concentration and the protein binding of the medication. Since antiepileptic drugs do not bind to protein in milk, the concentration of drug in milk will be approximately the same as the free plasma concentration. The higher the plasma-protein binding, the less drug that will be excreted in the milk. Phenytoin is very poorly absorbed from the infant gastrointestinal tract and tightly bound to plasma proteins; consequently, no detectable amounts of phenytoin are usually found in the plasma of breastfed infants whose mothers take phenytoin. The amount of phenobarbital obtained in breast milk can be significant, and some infants nursing from mothers on phenobarbital will have significant plasma concentrations of phenobarbital. Clinical symptoms such as poor suck, lethargy, and irritability may ensue. While low plasma concentrations of carbamazepine may be present in infants who are nursing, clinical symptoms appear to be minimal. The amount of exposure to valproate is minimal and rarely presents a problem.

G. Management

All women of childbearing potential should be told the risks associated with pregnancy. Decisions regarding antiepileptic drug therapy should be made before the woman becomes pregnant. If the woman has been seizure-free for a few years, the need for continued drugs should be reconsidered. If the woman is on polytherapy, attempts should be made to convert to monotherapy before she becomes pregnant. Monotherapy should be reduced to the lowest effective dose. All women contemplating pregnancy should be on folic acid, 2 to 4 mg/day.

All of the commonly used antiepileptic drugs are associated with both minor and major malformations. The drug of choice, therefore, is that antiepileptic which controls a woman's seizures without causing side effects. However, women with a family history of neural tube defects should probably avoid valproic acid and carbamazepine. During the pregnancy it is important that toxic and subtherapeutic concentrations should be avoided. Because of the increased clearance of antiepileptic drugs during pregnancy, it is frequently necessary for the dosages of antiepileptic drugs to be increased. If the patient experiences signs of toxicity in the face of apparent therapeutic drug levels, a free-phenytoin or valproate-plasma concentration determination may be useful.

An ultrasonographic evaluation should be performed to rule out spina bifida, cardiac anomalies, or a limb defect at 16 to 18 weeks. If ultrasound examination is not conclusive, amniocentesis should be performed, and alpha-fetoprotein levels obtained. Vitamin K_1 should be administered (20 mg/day), beginning 3 weeks before expected delivery until birth to prevent neonatal hemorrhage.

Good nutrition and adequate sleep are essential. The patient must avoid use of other medications except as directed by a physician. Smoking and the consumption of alcohol should be avoided, as this has been associated with fetal anomalies. Alcohol may also stimulate hepatic pathways, altering the metabolism of antiepileptic drugs, and, thus, altering the risk that malformations may occur.

Although the risks to the mother with epilepsy and her offspring are greater than the normal population, it is important to remember that approximately 90% of women with epilepsy have an uneventful pregnancy and normal infant.

II. THE ELDERLY

A. Epidemiology

The prevalence and cumulative incidence of epilepsy (Fig. 1-1) and the incidence of partial seizures (Fig. 1-2) increase dramatically in the elderly. The prevalence rate of active epilepsy (usually localization-related) is approximately 1.5% among persons 65 years of age and older. Approximately 10% of elderly nursing home residents receive an antiepileptic drug.

B. Etiology

Most seizures with onset after age 65 are caused by localization-related/symptomatic (partial, focal) seizures. The age-specific etiologies of these epilepsies are reviewed in Chapter 3 and Fig. 3-1. Cerebrovascular disease is the etiology in approximately 75% of seizures in the elderly. Seizures may occur at the time of stroke onset (10% to 20% of cases), or later as recurring seizures (5% to 20% of cases). Seizures may be particularly common after subarachnoid hemorrhages, in patients with seizures immediately after a cerebral infarction, and in patients with recurrent cerebral infarction. The risk of seizures in patients with Alzheimer's disease is 5 to 10 times that of the general population.

C. Diagnosis: Electroencephalography (EEG)

A number of normal patterns in the elderly can be mistaken for abnormalities suggesting epilepsy. These include: benign temporal delta transients of the elderly, frontally dominant rhythmic activity at onset of drowsiness, and electrocardiograph artifact caused by ventricular premature contractions (may appear to be temporal spikes). Medications and disease states also may alter the EEG in the elderly. See review of Klass and Brenner (4) for details.

D. Differential Diagnosis

Epilepsy frequently must be distinguished from syncope, transient ischemic attacks, and transient global amnesia in the elderly. These differential diagnoses are discussed in Chapter 9.

E. Management: Clinical Pharmacology

The absorption, distribution, biotransformation, excretion, drug interactions, and toxicology of antiepileptic drugs are all effected by age.

1. Absorption

Gastrointestinal motility, absorptive surface area, and splanchnic blood flow decreases and gastric PH increases with age. However, other factors such as concomitant food intake, concomitant therapy, and underlying disease have even greater importance in determining absorption. Overall, there are no consistent rules regarding how drug absorption will vary with age.

2. Distribution: Volume of Distribution

With increasing age, total body water and lean body mass decrease, while fat mass increases. This results in a decreased volume of distribution (and increased plasma concentration) of water-soluble drugs such as ethanol and caffeine. Conversely, there is an increased volume of distribution (and decreased plasma concentration) of lipid-soluble drugs, such as valproic acid and clonazepam.

3. Distribution: Protein Binding

Plasma albumin (principal drug-binding protein) concentration decreases by 5% to 10% in the elderly. This results in less protein binding and a higher free (unbound) fraction for drugs which are tightly bound to albumin. This, in turn, results in greater efficacy and toxicity for a given total plasma concentration of drug in the elderly. Phenytoin and valproic acid demonstrate this phenomenon.

4. Biotransformation

Hepatic mass and volume decrease by 15% to 20% between young and old adults. Decrease in clearance through cytochrome oxidase (cytochrome *P-450*) enzymes roughly correlates with decreased hepatic mass and volume for many (but not all) drugs metabolized by these enzymes. Carbamazepine, phenytoin, phenobarbital, and valproic acid exhibit this phenomenon. Unfortunately, the extent of slowed metabolism varies greatly among individuals and is difficult to predict.

5. Excretion

There is a 10% to 20% decrease in renal mass, blood flow, size and number of nephrons, and glomerular surface area between young and old adults. This is accompanied by a corresponding decrease in measures of renal function such as creatinine clearance and tubular excretory capacity, and decrease in clearance of drugs cleared by direct renal excretion, such as gabapentin and topiramate. Unlike hepatic biotransformation, renal excretion has a consistent and predictable decrease with age.

6. Drug Interactions

The elderly often take multiple types of drugs, putting them at risk for drug-drug interactions. Such interactions are particularly common when antiepileptic drugs metabolized by the hepatic cytochrome *P-450* system (carbamazepine, phenobarbital, phenytoin, primidone) are administered with each other, or with other types of drugs also metabolized by the cytochrome *P-450*. The reader is advised to consult the package insert or an appropriate pharmacy text/computer program before adding another drug to an antiepileptic drug or vice versa.

7. Toxicity

Certain toxicities of antiepileptic drugs appear to be more severe at a given free or total plasma concentration of certain drugs in the elderly, when compared with younger patients. These toxicities and drugs include: sedation and behavioral changes (clonazepam, phenobarbital, primidone), tremor (valproic acid), and hyponatremia (carbamazepine).

8. Consequences of Polypharmacy

The elderly often take multiple drugs. The elderly constitute 12% of the population and consume 25% of prescription drugs. The average elderly resident in a long-term facility is taking 5 to 6 prescription drugs. This polypharmacy puts the elderly at risk for drug toxicity and drug-drug interactions. Side effects and interactions of prescription drugs account for 17% of hospitalizations in the elderly, vs 3% of hospitalizations in the overall population.

F. Management: Drug Selection

Most seizures in the elderly are of the localization-related (partial) type. Carbamazepine and phenytoin have been the drugs of choice for localization-related seizures, based upon comparative studies of older antiepileptic drugs performed with nonelderly adults. Furthermore, phenobarbital, primidone and valproic acid all have toxicity problems in the elderly (see previously).

The ideal antiepileptic drug for the elderly would have minimal protein binding, minimal oxidative metabolism, and minimal neurotoxicity. Carbamazepine and phenytoin fail all three of these criteria, while the newer drugs gabapentin and lamotrigine pass. Gabapentin has the added advantages of no drug interactions and no serious toxicity. Gabapentin and lamotrigine are the drugs of choice for use as adjuncts to carbamazepine and phenytoin (FDA-approved indications). Gabapentin and/or lamotrigine may become initial drugs of choice for partial seizures in the elderly (not yet on FDA-approved indication), based upon the criteria for an ideal antiepileptic drug described previously in this paragraph. Because gabapentin is excreted entirely by the kidney, gabapentin dosage in elderly patients with a creatinine clearance value of less than 60 ml/min, should be reduced following guidelines contained in the package insert.

REFERENCES

1. Cloyd JC. Clinical pharmacology of antiepileptic drugs in the elderly: practical applications. *Consult Pharmac* 1995;10:9–15.
2. Delgado-Escueta AV, Janz D, Beck-Mannagetta G. Pregnancy and teratogenesis in epilepsy. *Neurology* 1992;(suppl 5):42.
3. Engel J, Pedley TA, eds. *Epilepsy: a comprehensive textbook.* Philadelphia: Lippincott–Raven, 1997, Chapters 106, 187–192.
4. Klass DW, Brenner RP. Electroencephalography of the elderly. *J Clin Neurophysiol* 1995;12:116–131.
5. Kotila M, Waltimo O. Epilepsy after stroke. *Epilepsia* 1992;33:495–498.
6. Morrell MJ. Hormones, reproductive health, and epilepsy. In: Wyllie E, ed. *The treatment of epilepsy: principles and practice,* 2nd ed. Baltimore: Williams and Wilkins, 1997.
7. Parker BM, Vestal RE. Pharmacokinetics of anti-convulsant drugs in the elderly. In: Wyllie E, ed. *The treatment of epilepsy: principles and practice.* 2nd ed. Baltimore: Williams and Wilkins, 1997.
8. Ramsay RE, Rowan AJ. *Epilepsy and seizures in the elderly.* New York: Butterworth, 1996.
9. Schener ML. Drug treatment in the elderly. In: Engel J, Pedley TA, eds. *Epilepsy: a comprehensive textbook.* Philadelphia: Lippincott–Raven, 1997.
10. So EL, Annegers JF, Hanser WA, et al. Population-based study of seizure disorders after cerebral infarction. *Neurology* 1996;46:350–355.
11. Willmore LJ: The effect of age on pharmacokinetics of antiepileptic drugs. *Epilepsia* 1995;36 (suppl 5): 514–521.
12. Yerby MS. Treatment of epilepsy during pregnancy. In: Wyllie E, ed. *The treatment of epilepsy: principles and practice,* 2nd ed. Baltimore: Williams and Wilkins, 1997.
13. Yerby MS, Collins SD. Pregnancy: mother and child. In: Engel J, Pedley TA, eds. *Epilepsy: a comprehensive textbook.* Philadelphia: Lippincott–Raven, 1997.

COUNSELING

I. COUNSELING ISSUES FOR CHILDREN

A. Activities

While children with epilepsy are at increased risk for injury, limitations on activities should be relatively few. When restrictions are excessive they may lead to significant psychological difficulties with impaired self-esteem.

Childhood is filled with inherent risks, and the child with epilepsy is only at a minimally greater risk than before the seizures began. It is not possible to make guidelines that can be applied to all children with epilepsy, because seizure type, duration, and frequency are factors that may affect the number of restrictions.

Restrictions may also vary over the course of the disorder. Restrictions should be more stringent during the first 2 to 3 months after onset of the disorder, until the physician and family are in agreement that further seizures are unlikely, and for 2 to 3 months after discontinuing antiepileptic medication. In children with persistent, recurrent seizures restrictions usually remain the same.

Parents must be particularly careful around *water*. Children with epilepsy are at higher risk for drowning than children without epilepsy, either in a bathtub or during recreational swimming. Young children should never be left alone in the bathtub, even for a few seconds. Older children should be encouraged to use a shower and reminded not to lock the bathroom door when showering. Unsupervised swimming should never occur.

All children should avoid *open fires*, *hot stoves*, or *ovens*, and *dangerous machinery*. Parents must assume that a seizure could occur at any time and should avoid allowing a child to be in a situation where a seizure could be deadly. For example, children should not stand near the platform of subway or train stations.

There should be very few restrictions of *recreational activities*. Activities in which the child is high off the ground, such as rock or rope climbing should be discouraged. While bike riding can be pursued safely in most children, it should be avoided in children with frequent seizures in whom there is impairment of consciousness. Skating, rollerblading, and skateboarding should be restricted only in children with frequent seizures. Even in children with well-controlled epilepsy, these activities should not occur on busy streets. Obviously, sky diving and scuba diving should be prohibited.

The child with epilepsy should be encouraged to participate in *organized sports*. While some physicians restrict contact sports in the belief that head trauma can precipitate seizures, there is no evidence that patients with epilepsy are at higher risk for seizures following minor head injury. Children who have a regular exercise program may actually have fewer seizures and side effects than children who are sedentary.

Parents of young children are often terrified that the child will have an undetected seizure and die during *sleep*. Having the child sleep in the same room of the parents may be appropriate for the first few months after diagnosis. The parents should also be instructed to purchase an intercom that can be turned on and placed in the child's room so they can be alerted by any crying or an abnormal breathing pattern. Infants or young children should avoid soft or restricting sleeping surfaces.

Caregivers other than the parents should be told that the child has epilepsy and be given a description of the seizure, along with first-aid measures. Since seizures can be extremely frightening, babysitters should be chosen with care. Local epilepsy support groups often have a list of experienced babysitters.

Children who are at risk for prolonged seizures present additional problems when the *family travels* or visits remote areas where medical care may not be readily available. Before traveling, parents should inquire as to the closest medical facility that would deal with a child with epilepsy. It is also recommended that the parents be given instruction in administering rectal diazepam in case a prolonged seizure ensues. A test dose under the supervision of a nurse or physician is recommended before doing this in an emergency situation.

B. Television and Video Games

Rarely, children will have a seizure while watching television, playing an electronic screen game, or using a computer. Most of these children will have a photoconvulsive response on the EEG. Television, computer and video games should be restricted only when there is a consistent relationship between watching television or playing video games and seizures. Parents will often erroneously blame video game playing or television watching for the seizure, even when the seizure occurs at a later time. The parents must be informed that if television or the video game is responsible for the seizure, it will occur during the time the activity is occurring.

C. School

Children with epilepsy are at significant risk for a variety of problems involving cognition and behavior. The distribution of IQ scores are skewed toward lower values, and the number of children requiring special education services vary from 10% to 33%. Behavioral and psychiatric disorders in children with epilepsy are also higher than in the normal population, with surveys demonstrating that the prevalence of psychiatric disease is 2 to 4 times greater among children with epilepsy than control subjects. While the cognitive and behavioral abnormalities may often be explained by the etiologic factors responsible for the epilepsy, there is evidence that some children with poorly controlled epilepsy have progressive declines of IQ on serial intelligence tests, and behavioral and psychiatric deterioration over time. Whether this decline is secondary to antiepileptic medications, progression of the underlying encephalopathy responsible for the seizures, or the seizures per se, is not certain.

There are a number of factors that place the child at increased risk for cognitive impairment: an early age of seizure onset, intractable seizures, and polytherapy. The etiology of the epilepsy is also important. Children with symptomatic epilepsy are at higher risk for cognitive impairment than those with idiopathic epilepsy.

It is important for the physician and the child's teachers be aware of these potential difficulties since they should be addressed as soon as they are identified. The child may benefit from special education resources, such as speech, physical, and occupational therapy. In children with learning difficulties, it is important to avoid drug toxicity. Polytherapy and treatment with barbiturates and benzodiazepines should be avoided when possible.

School personnel working with the child should be informed of the child's condition and the treatment plan. Little is gained from trying to keep the diagnosis secret and epilepsy "off the record." Teachers can provide the physician with assessment regarding seizure frequency and drug side effects and serve as advocates for the child. Since children with seizures may be the subject of ridicule by classmates, informed teachers can educate the class about the disorder and dispel many of the myths that accompany the diagnosis.

II. COUNSELING ISSUES FOR ADULTS

A. Pregnancy
See Chapter 13.

B. Risk of Epilepsy in First-Degree Relatives
Patients with epilepsy often ask if relatives (especially children) have an increased risk of epilepsy. The epilepsy syndromes are divided by etiology into symptomatic and idiopathic types (see Chapter 1). There is little or no increased risk for epilepsy in first-degree relatives of patients with symptomatic epilepsies. First-degree relatives of patients with idiopathic epilepsies have an increased risk (2- to 3-fold on average) of epilepsy. The increased risk of idiopathic epilepsy in relatives of patients with idiopathic epilepsy decreases with age; risk is not increased at age 35 or older. See Ottman et al. (6) for further information.

C. Driving
Driving privileges must balance the risk of a seizure while driving to the patient and the public against the other considerable negative effects of loss of driving privileges to the patient. Persons with active seizure disorders must be made known to the state registry of motor vehicles and have driving privileges suspended until their seizures are controlled.

In most states, it is the patient's responsibility to report their active seizure condition to the registry of motor vehicles. It is a breach of patient confidentiality for the physician to make such a report. In a few states, the physician must report the patient to a state authority.

Adequate seizure control can be determined several ways. Most states require a patient be seizure-free on medication for a specified period of time (usually 3 to 12 months). The patient may then re-apply for driving privileges. Such an application usually requires a letter from the patient's physician. Other states have a medical board which determines driving eligibility on an individual basis. Some states use a combination of the two methods.

Because state laws are variable and changing, the physician is best advised to contact state authorities in his/her state regarding current regulations. The physician must advise the patient of current state regulations regarding driving. This advice should be given in writing to the patient as a form letter and distribution to the patient recorded in the record. Note that regulations for operation of buses and/or large trucks usually are different and more restrictive than regulations for operation of a personal automobile.

The following are suggestions for helping patients deal with life without driving privileges: (1) public transportation; (2) car pools, (3) find a person (e.g., student, retiree) willing to serve as a driver.

D. Insurance

1. Health and Life

Some medical and life insurance companies either penalize persons with epilepsy or won't insure them at all. Many companies offer limited coverage, usually excluding pre-existing epilepsy. The following advice is offered: (a) check any health or life insurance plan to be certain epilepsy-related events are covered; (b) employer group insurance plans tend to be less selective and more likely to cover pre-existing epilepsy; (c) determine if the patient is eligible for Medicare, Medicaid, or veterans benefits or state-administered free medication programs; and (d) most states have a state insurance regulatory agency which can provide advice.

2. Driving

Driving insurance may be difficult to obtain. Some states have a special "pool" providing driving insurance to persons perceived to be a greater risk.

E. Employment

The question of seizures may come up when a person with epilepsy seeks employment. The Americans with Disability Act (ADA, private employers) and Federal Rehabilitation Act (federal agencies and contractors) prohibit employers from discriminating against persons with a disability who could perform the job with "reasonable accommodations." Persons with epilepsy can perform most jobs and should be excluded only when having a seizure would pose a danger to the person or co-workers (e.g., driving, operating dangerous machinery, working at heights). Persons with epilepsy should: (a) learn about any job they are applying for before the interview; (b) complete the application process if they are qualified; and (c) take action if discriminated against. The federal Department of Labor, state agencies for disabled persons, and the Epilepsy Foundation of America are good resources for employment-related advice.

F. Income Assistance

Persons with reduced ability to work because of disability may qualify for Supplemental Security Income (SSI) under the Social Security Administration or veterans benefits (health services and/or income) under the Department of Veterans Affairs. The eligibility requirements are complex. Assistance may be obtained from: (a) references at the end of this chapter; (b) social work agencies; (c) the Social Security Administration; (d) the Department of Veterans Affairs Assistance Hot Line (800-827-1000); and (e) veterans groups (e.g., Disabled American Veterans).

G. When All Else Fails

Local epilepsy groups, the Epilepsy Foundation of America, and other advocacy groups often can lead the person with epilepsy to the right resource. Groups representing other disabilities (e.g., developmental disabilities, head injury) may have useful information. The state attorney general's office is responsible for protecting citizens' civil and consumer rights and can offer advice in these areas. Persons with epilepsy should ask forcefully for assistance and seek the resources they need.

REFERENCES

1. Engel J, Pedley TA, eds. *Epilepsy: a comprehensive textbook.* Philadelphia: Lippincott–Raven, 1997, Chapters 206–212.
2. Farwell JR, Dodril CB, Batzel LW. Neuropsychological abilities of children with epilepsy. *Epilepsia* 1985;26:395–400.
3. Fraser RT. Overview: Social issues. In: Engel J, Pedley TA, eds. *Epilepsy: a comprehensive textbook.* Philadelphia: Lippincott–Raven, 1997.
4. Hansotta P, Broste SK. Epilepsy and traffic safety. *Epilepsia* 1993;34:852–858.
5. Holmes GL. The long-term effects of seizures on the developing brain: clinical and laboratory issues. *Brain Dev* 1991;13:393–409.

6. Lehman C. Legal aspects of epilepsy. In: Wyllie E, ed. *The treatment of epilepsy: principles and practice,* 2nd ed. Baltimore: Williams and Wilkins, 1997.

7. Moshe SL, Pellock JM, Salon MC. *The Parke-Davis manual on epilepsy: useful tips that help you get the best out of life.* New York: MSF Group, 1993.

8. Ottman R, Annegers JF, Risch N, et al. Relations of genetic and environmental factors in etiology of epilepsy. *Ann Neurol* 1996;39:442–449.

9. Quirk JA, Fish DR, Smith SJ, et al. First seizures associated with playing electronic screen games: a community-based study in Great Britain. *Ann Neurol* 1995;37L:733–737.

10. Shaw EB. Resources available to the patient with epilepsy. In: Browne TR, Feldman RG, eds. *Epilepsy: diagnosis and management.* Boston: Little Brown, 1983.

11. Wyllie E, ed. *The treatment of epilepsy: principles and practice,* 2nd ed. Baltimore: Williams and Wilkins, 1997, Chapters 84–92.

APPENDIX I

Conversion Table for Antiepileptic Drug Plasma Concentration Determinations

WEIGHT-PER-VOLUME CONVERSIONS

10 micrograms per milliliter (µg/ml) = 10 milligrams per liter (mg/L) = 1.0 milligrams per 100 milliliters (mg/100 ml) = 1.0 milligrams per deciliter (mg/dl)

WEIGHT-PER-VOLUME TO MOLAR CONVERSIONS
DRUG CONVERSION FACTOR
(µg/ml to µmoles)

Carbamazepine	4.232
Clonazepam	3.168
Ethosuximide	7.083
Gabapentin	5.840
Lamotrigine	3.927
Phenobarbital	4.306
Phenytoin	3.964
Primidone	4.581
Topiramate	2.947
Valproic acid	6.934
Vigabatrin	7.742

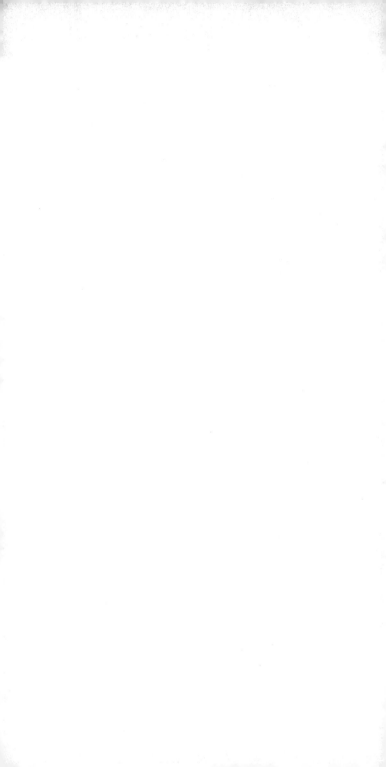

Index

Page numbers followed by *f* indicate figures; those followed by *t* indicate tables.